any medication you might be taking. This book is not intended to be a substitute for professional medical advice, diagnosis, or treatment.

Building Lean Muscle Mass

- **Clean Bulking Tips**
- **Women & Weight Training**
- **Back**
- **Biceps**
- **Calf**
- **Hamstrings**
- **Neck**
- **Quadriceps**
- **Shoulder**
- **Triceps**

Introduction

After several years of working in fitness centers and gyms, the one thing that amazes me is seeing people in these locations who couldn't tell you the difference between their triceps and their hamstrings (if you currently don't know the difference you will by the end of this book). Why spend all that time working on your health and fitness just to have no idea what you are doing or even why? Stop simply going through the motions. Learning is part of the experience.

I want this book to be used as a tool to help you understand the principles of exercise, proper nutrition, and just about everything you'd need to know during your journey. Too often people work out for endless hours each week not getting the results they desired. This book will help teach the basics as well as get into detail on the various topics covered including exercises, muscles of the body, diet, nutrition, and much more.

When this book is read in its entirety, you should clearly understand exactly what you are doing when you work out and how to create workouts and diets to achieve the results you want. You will also get varies tips on how to achieve your results faster by setting yourself up for success.

<u>Let's start off with some simple questions…</u>

Do you know all the muscles you hit when doing a specific exercise?

Do you know what exercises hit what muscle groups?

Do you know what you need to eat in order to get the results you desire?

Do you know what supplements you need to help put on lean muscle mass?

Once you stop seeing results, do you know how to break through plateaus?

If you answered "no" to any of those questions then this book will help you understand not only the topics you inquire about, but also give you further knowledge on topics that you thought you knew everything about, but were missing vital pieces of information.

Clean Bulking Tips

When beach weather starts to fade and the summer cut is finally coming to a close, that's when the fun begins. It's time to bulk gentleman (and ladies…)! For those of you just starting out, this is probably all new to you and you really don't understand the concept of cutting and bulking and why things happen during certain times of the year.

For most, fall/winter is the time to bulk and put on lean muscle mass. If they add a little fat during this time, so be it, not a big deal. Most people will be wearing a lot of long sleeve sweatshirt types of clothing; therefore, they can hide whatever fat they might gain if any. This isn't a time to completely let yourself go though.

Then come spring/summer, that's the time to cut and drop the fat that you might have gained during the cold months to show off the new lean mass you added. Not to mention, most people go to the beach or go on vacation these months so it naturally makes sense to diet and hit some cardio during this time. Bulking during this time will have you looking slightly heavier/bloated than if you were cutting. Any fat gains associated with bulking will be apparent especially when in a bathing suit.

Now onto the good stuff! We all start from scratch. We aren't placed on this earth to know everything without learning about it first. So here I am to the rescue! The rest of this section is especially for the new guys (or gals) who need some tips on how to effectively bulk. The following are ten tips (in no particular order) to help you on your way to packing on some muscle.

1) Food

Here is a compilation of things that you should consider having on your grocery list (you may pick and choose the foods in those categories that you like):

<u>Proteins</u>

- Beef Tenderloin
- Boneless, Skinless Chicken Breast
 -Egg Whites or Eggs
- Extra Lean Ground Beef or Ground Round
- Eye of Round
- Fish
- Flank Steak
- Ground Turkey, Turkey Breast Slices or Cutlets (fresh sources, not deli cuts)
- Protein Powder
- Ribeye Steaks or Roast
- Shrimp
- Top Round Steaks or Roast

- Top Sirloin
- Top Loin
- Tuna (fresh cut or tuna in can/package with water, not in oil)

Complex Carbs

- Beans (Black, Kidney, Pinto)
- Brown Rice
- Cream of Wheat
- Garbanzo Beans
- Green Peas
- Legumes
- Lentils
- Lima Beans
- Multi-Grain Hot Cereal
- Oat Bran Cereal
- Oatmeal (Old Fashioned or Quick Oats)
- Pasta
- Potatoes (Red or Baking)
- Quinoa
- Rice (White, Jasmine, Wild)
- Sweet Potatoes
- Yams
- Whole-Grains (Bread or Cereal)

Fibrous Carbs

- Asparagus
- Bell Peppers
- Broccoli
- Brussels Sprouts

- Carrots
- Cauliflower
- Celery
- Cucumber
- Egg Plant
- Green Beans
- Green Leafy Lettuce (Green Leaf, Red Leaf, Romaine)
- Kale
- Mushrooms
- Onions
- Peppers (Green or Red)
- Spaghetti Squash
- Spinach
- String Beans
- Zucchini

Fruits

- Apples
- Bananas
- Blueberries
- Grapefruit
- Grapes
- Kiwis
- Oranges
- Papayas
- Raspberries
- Strawberries
- Tomatoes

Healthy Fats

- Fatty Cold-Water Fish (Bluefish, Mackerel, Mullet, Sablefish, Salmon)
- Monounsaturated Oils (Canola, Olive, Peanut)
- More Fish (Anchovy, Herring, Lake Trout, Sardines, Tuna)
- Natural Almond Butter
- Natural Peanut Butter
- Nuts (Almonds, Peanuts, Pistachios, Walnuts)
- Polyunsaturated Oils (Corn, Cottonseed, Safflower, Soybean, Sunflower)
- Seeds (Flaxseeds, Pumpkin, Sunflower)

Dairy & Eggs

- Eggs (Whole)
- Low-Fat Cottage Cheese
- Low-Fat Yogurt
- Low or Non-Fat Milk

While bulking you want to eat more calories (more than maintenance) and because of this, you might need to eat more often and/or eat more at each meal. Each meal should consist of protein, carbs, and fats. It doesn't have to be anything big; it could be something as simple as an apple with peanut butter if that's all you can fit into a small timeframe between class or meetings at work depending on if you are a student or working professional. Meal frequency and timing isn't something to pay much attention too so long as you're getting in your daily caloric intake. In the past, it was thought that if you ate 5-7 small meals during the day that you were able to keep your metabolism revving all day long, but science has since debunked that.

You should also be striving for around 1 gram of protein per pound of bodyweight you have. I'd recommend striving for 1 gram to start with and see how your body responds but you can also see results from backing it off to 0.7 grams per pound of body weight. The increase in protein from where you probably are right now is necessary to feed the muscles the nutrients they need to repair and grow. Protein is made up of amino acids which are the building blocks of protein and essentially muscle. So, if you weigh 150 pounds, the 1 gram figure would have you hitting 150 grams of protein per day.

Here's a little secret that I love to use myself and share with others. Tracking how much you eat all day can seem pretty tedious. What I would recommend doing is to download the MyFitnessPal app on your smartphone. You can then input all of your information and it will spit out how many calories you need to be eating in order to hit your goal. You can also change the macros as well to ensure you are getting your 1 gram of protein per pound of body weight each day.

The app itself then allows you to scan the barcode of the foods you eat which is then recognized. All you have to do is put in the serving size you ate. If you don't have a barcode on the item, you can search for it within the app and more than likely you will find exactly what you're looking for. Date night? No problem, the app also has many restaurants as well as fast food places that you can find through the search feature. All you have to do is enter the foods you ate at the given location and it will do all the rest for you.

Yes, using MyFitnessPal will make you weigh out your food, but if you want to see results and ensure you aren't way off with your diet, it's a necessary evil.

2) Supplements

Supplements are truly just as it is defined—a supplement to "something". In this case, it would be both macronutrients and micronutrients. Supplements should never replace whole food options unless necessary to hit any missing pieces of your nutrition throughout your day. I'm not a fan of taking everything under the sun and for that reason, I have just a few staples that everyone should consider.

Below is a list of supplements which are great during any time of the year, including while bulking. Note, I do not recommend supplementation for anyone under the age of 18, and I cannot stress enough the fact that supplementation should never be a replacement for good proper nutrition.

<u>Whey Protein (Concentrate or Isolate)</u>

Protein is the building block for muscle. Without it, you won't make the gains you are looking for. You can use whey protein at any time of the day. There are many different brands and flavors out there, find one that suits your taste buds and isn't overly priced.

You can use it pre-workout, post-workout, as a snack, or add some fruit with natural peanut butter and throw it in the blender with some ice cubes and use it as a meal replacement if you need something quick on the go and can't get in a real food meal. It is a quick and easy way to help you get in your daily protein intake should you find you can't eat enough during the day to hit your numbers.

Whey protein in the form of a protein shake is also ideal post-workout as it is quicker to be absorbed (due to it being in liquid form) when compared to a whole food option that would need to get broken down before being shuttled through the bloodstream to help muscles recover.

<u>Casein Protein</u>

Casein protein is the best protein you can get if you are looking for a slow release of nutrients. This particular type of protein is a slow-digesting, which means it slowly breaks down the protein and nutrients and releases them into your system over a span of around 6-8 hours. This protein comes in especially handy before bed when compared to a straight whey isolate product.

If you get a blended whey protein that includes casein (which many of them do), there is no reason to purchase a strict casein protein product. Simply use the same product if it falls into the whey protein category mentioned above.

<u>Multivitamin & Mineral</u>

It is a necessity to purchase a good multivitamin & mineral. You need to get proper vitamins and minerals, which you can't get from food alone. A multivitamin/mineral is essential to help with everyday activities and give you exactly what your body needs to maintain a healthy lifestyle. Micronutrients are overlooked by many, yet is something everyone should pay close attention to.

Through diet alone, we generally wouldn't be able to get the daily recommended value of certain micronutrients because of the sheer amount of food that would need to be consumed, so for that reason, a good multivitamin/mineral should be a staple in your supplementation regimen.

Creatine

Creatine will help you not only recover faster, but it will help you gain some lean muscle mass quicker. Creatine is one of the most widely studied supplements out on the market today. There are no harmful effects from creatine and it can be used safely before and after workouts. There is no need to do a loading phase or cycle creatine.

With the many forms of creatine out on the market, I would recommend starting with the one that was used in the most studies—monohydrate. Some individuals are non-responders to monohydrate but for most people, it will work just fine and happens to be the least expensive. If you find you're a non-responder, consider trying CEE or Creatine HCl.

Fish Oil

Fish oil gives you EFA's (essential fatty acids), which are the "good fats" that we all need. Fatty acids are a necessity, which most people don't understand. They are important for cellular, heart, and metabolic health. We do not get enough "good fats" in our diet each day so supplementing with fish oil is very beneficial.

Look for a product that contains docosahexaenoic acid (DHA) and eicosapentaenoic acid (EPA) as they have several health benefits. This duo may help prevent memory loss, may improve cholesterol levels, can help improve focus, helps to maintain strong bones, may support healthy brain function, and may give you a better sense of well-being as well as boosting your mood.

3) Compound Movements

Compound movements are what make you grow better than any other type of movement. It's with good reason that it's recommended that those just starting out in the gym should master compound movements before working in any other type of exercise movements. Isolation movements are more for the shaping of muscles rather than jacking up the growth hormones in your body and gaining some serious mass.

Compound movements are the squat, deadlift, barbell press, military press, and similar movements that involve several muscle groups being activated in order to complete the movement or exercise. These movements are considered the foundation of putting on lean muscle mass while bulking.

4) Rest

It's a fact that you don't grow while in the gym. You grow while you rest after your workout. Sure, when you have a nice hard pump in the gym and your muscles are swollen and look larger you think you're getting bigger and bigger each set. You are incorrect. That nice pump that we all long for is only temporary. Your muscles become engorged with blood giving the larger appearance. After about an hour those effects start to diminish and you will be about the same size as you were before you stepped into the gym that day.

You need to rest your muscles and get adequate sleep at night to help increase growth hormones in your body which in turn help you gain lean muscle mass. Strive to get no less than 8 hours of sleep a night. Anything less and you will be cutting yourself short with your gains.

5) Post-Workout Meal

Post-workout meals are very important and should be consumed within 45 minutes after your workout. You can think of it as an old coal train. You throw a whole bunch of coal in to start the train and then you stop giving it coal, what eventually happens? The train stops. Same goes with your body. The food you eat pre-workout gets used as fuel for the body during exercise. Then as your workout comes to an end, the fuel has surely run out and it will be starving for more to function and grow.

If you don't feed your body, it can't grow. And it is especially needed post-workout because that is when your body absorbs nutrients best. Your body is literally starving for nutrients at the end of your workout and if you don't feed it then it simply can't repair itself and grow properly.

In the post-workout meal, you should be taking in around 20-40 grams of protein. Add in double that amount of carbohydrates (40-80 grams). Have the carbohydrate source coming from simple sources rather than complex carbohydrates so they can help spike insulin and shuttle the nutrients to the muscles faster.

This book will also touch on supplements a little bit later in the book to give you an idea of how to keep money in your pocket when picking out the best type of supplements to fit your needs.

6) Keep Cardio to a Minimum

This one isn't rocket science and you don't need a Ph.D. to understand. Obviously, when you do cardio, you use up fuel (calories). Calories are what you need to grow. You take away calories, you take away potential gains. Now I'm not saying to stop cardio altogether, because you don't need to and continuing some cardio is great for the cardiovascular system as a whole along with health benefits.

Cardio is actually a good way to keep from putting on body fat during a bulking phase and an excellent way to keep the heart-healthy. Cardio also increases your appetite so you will be able to down some extra calories to make up for the loss you experienced during your workout.

You can get away with doing some low-intensity cardio without losing lean mass gains so do not be afraid to do cardio while bulking. I recommend a low-intensity cardio workout such as a walk outside or on the treadmill.

7) Increase Your Calories

In order to gain weight (muscle), you must increase your calories. This does not mean you can eat McDonald's or Wendy's every meal since you would be increasing your calories. You could do that, but I wouldn't recommend it unless you want to look like a blimp. An easy way to do this (especially if you are stuck at the same weight) is to track your calories.

When you find out how many calories you are eating which maintains your weight, add 250-500 calories each day and by the end of the week see if you gained any weight. Don't forget that 3,500 calories are equal to one pound. So theoretically, if you increased your calories by 500 each day for a week you should gain a pound (this will not be all lean muscle mass).

Now let me explain something to you, this isn't as easy as you may think. You can't just eat some Twinkies or eat a cake. You still need to be eating clean to ensure you don't gain fat. Yes, during your bulking phase, you will gain some fat. But do not get worried about this unless you are gaining a lot of fat in which case you need to look at your diet and clean it up a little. It would be a smart idea for you to write down your weight once a week on the same day and at the same time. This will help with the accuracy of your results and see how you are progressing. You can also get your body fat measured once a week to see how much fat you are gaining if any at all. Like I already mentioned, if you are gaining a lot of fat, re-evaluate your diet.

8) Water

Water is a key no matter what you are trying to accomplish. Staying hydrated increases protein synthesis so you will make better use of the protein you ingest. Water is also a good way to stay hydrated without adding all the sugary drinks like soda and tea.

Strive for at least a gallon of water a day. If you sweat a lot during your workout you definitely should be striving for more than a gallon a day. An easy way to track your water intake is to carry around a gallon jug wherever you go or at a minimum use water from a gallon jug and fill your glass/cup from that same jug every time your glass/cup is empty. When it's empty, you know you got your gallon in. This is a great way to track how much water you are taking in each day. If you find the gallon jug is empty before the end of the day, at that point you can refill and keep going. Water also keeps your metabolism revving due to the oxygen content in the water.

9) Training

Most people have the mentality that more is better. This is not the case with training. Most of the time the people who have that mindset are overtraining and in turn minimizing their gains. Depending on your exercise level, you could train smartly with 3-5 days in the gym depending on how you structure your workouts. You want to keep your workouts short and intense. This means that you should ideally keep your workouts less than 1 hour. Anything more and you are lowering your natural testosterone levels, which you don't want to do.

The key is to experiment and find out what training style works best for your body. Some people respond very well to lower rep sets while others find higher reps sets are the way to go. Some people can get away with a low number of sets (6-8) for each body part while some people need to complete many sets to get results (12+). I would actually recommend starting with lower sets, evaluate your progress and adjust it accordingly. If you find you aren't growing with the number of sets you are doing, gradually increase the sets and see how you respond to that.

When it comes down to it, there really is no one way to train. Everyone is different. The fun part is trying new things to see what works best for you. If building the body of your dreams and improving your health were easy, then everyone would look good and never get sick. It takes hard work and determination. Keep training hard and never be afraid to switch things up. Hitting the muscle differently is what sparks new growth and is what I'm sure everyone is trying to accomplish.

10) Have Fun!

For most of us, fitness isn't our full-time job and what pays the bills. And for the majority of us, that is a good thing. The determination and hard work needed to improve your health and physique aren't for the faint of heart. In order to stick with your exercise program, you need to find something that motivates you and go with it.

Set some short and long-term goals for yourself and check on your progress and re-evaluate things if needed. Make things fun, try new things. You do not want to dread going to the gym every day. By evaluating your progress and seeing the improvements, that should be enough to make you want to keep going. Sure, there are days where everything around you is going wrong and you really don't feel like going to the gym, but once you are there everything changes. The weights don't complain; they don't yell at you. The treadmill doesn't remind you that you have tons of work that needs to be done at home. It's a great way to release stress and something that you can do just for you.

Fitness isn't just a weekly or monthly thing. Fitness is a lifestyle. Where it takes you, no one knows. But what do you have to lose by having fun in the process? Living the fitness lifestyle is a great way to stay healthy and achieve the body you always wanted.

Women & Weight Training

Let's face it, how many women do you know who say they won't step foot in a weight room because they think they will get big and bulky? If you're a female reading this, maybe that's something you personally think?   I'm sure everyone knows someone who uses this as an excuse. Sure, women can get muscular like men… if they use anabolic steroids. Other than that, the answer is simply no. Women do not produce enough testosterone to build muscle at the same rate as men. It is physically impossible for them to get big, bulky, and extremely muscular to the point of where they are as big as some of the muscle heads in the gym. Can women be stronger than men?   Absolutely! There are plenty of women out there who work out that can out-lift a good portion of the male population.

Women who want to look healthier by either putting on some lean muscle or by losing some stubborn fat shouldn't fear grabbing a pair of dumbbells or getting under a barbell. For the women who are already in the gym and telling the guys to quit hogging the bench or squat rack, good for you! More power to you. For those who only see what a weight room looks like from the cardio room, shame on you! There is nothing to be afraid of in the weight room. The guys in the gym won't make fun of you for using lighter weights. Most guys in the gym are there minding their own business trying to fit a workout into their busy schedule just like you. Who knows, you might just find that you can lift just as much as some of the guys!

In fact, women can do the same workout that men do (with the total weight lifted being the only difference)—AND the same amount of reps and sets. I actually recommend that women train like men and push themselves every time they train with weights. There is no use going to the gym and cutting your progress short by selecting weights that don't push your body and muscles to change.

Doing just cardio is ok, but you risk losing some lean muscle mass. I know what some of you are thinking... I want to look thinner so I'm fine losing whatever I need to in order to look that way. In actuality, if you skip the weights and just stick with cardio and lose muscle mass, you will actually be slowing down your metabolism. Obviously slowing down your metabolism will make you burn fewer calories and will stunt your weight loss progress. Muscle burns more calories than fat. This ultimately raises your basal metabolic rate (BMR). Your BMR is how many calories you would burn if you did nothing all day and basically lay in bed.

<u>Here is a formula to help you figure out your BMR (English version):</u>

Women:
BMR = 655 + (4.35 x weight in pounds) + (4.7 x height in inches) – (4.7 x age in years)

Men:
BMR = 66 + (6.23 x weight in pounds) + (12.7 x height in inches) – (6.8 x age in years)

<u>Let's break down some of the benefits women achieve from weight training:</u>

- Become stronger
- More energy
- Burn more calories/fat
- Tone muscles
- Feel better
- Look better
- Decrease the risk of coronary disease
- Prevent and fight osteoporosis
- Improve balance
- And more!

The Back

Anatomy of the Back

The Lats:

The largest muscle of your back is by far the lats. The latissimus dorsi starts all the way up at the upper end of the humerus and runs all the way down to the pelvic girdle. The lats function is to pull the arm down towards the pelvis.

The Traps:

Another powerful muscle of the back is the trapezius. The traps run all the way down the upper section of the spinal cord, connecting to the bony part of the scapula (shoulder blade) called the acromion and attaches to the middle of your back. The traps have a couple of main functions including scapular adduction (bringing the shoulder blades together), scapular depression (pulling the shoulder blades down), and scapular elevation (shrugging). This is also covered under the "Neck Building" section.

Smaller Muscles:

There are also some smaller muscles that aid in the movement of the back such as the teres major and the rhomboids. The teres major is found at the outside edge of the shoulder blade and attaches all the way up at the humerus. The main role of the teres major is to bring the arm towards your back.

The rhomboids are found on the spinal column and they attach to the middle of the shoulder blade. The rhomboids are used to bring the shoulder blades together.

There are also a whole bunch of little muscles in the back that run along your spine. There are the erector spinae, which includes the longissimus, spinalis, and the iliocostalis. The erector spinae is a group of muscles that are in and support the spine as well as extend the spine. The erector spinae muscles are attached to the vertebrae, pelvis, and also to the ribs.

Different Parts of the Back

Different exercises hit different parts of the back. For instance, doing wide grip pulldowns targets the outer back while doing close grip rows targets the middle of the back.

It's important to hit all parts of the back to create overall back development. The last thing you want is imbalances with your back muscles. To create a nice V-taper down to your waist you need overall development starting from your traps and working all the way down to the bottom of your lats. By creating a fully developed back, you can still have a waist larger than you want and still have it appear like your waist is tiny. Hitting the lats will help widen your back while hitting the middle of your back help pull out details and help create overall thickness.

Bodybuilding is all about muscular development and creating an illusion that makes you look larger than you really are, weight isn't as large of a factor as many assume. Weight comes more into play when someone wants to train to be a powerlifter. The use of the term "bodybuilder" will be used loosely as many perceive the term to be associated with the enormous physiques that many see on competitive stages yet for our use in this book it will be used for anyone looking to build their overall muscles and physique without needing to step on stage.

Different Back Exercises

- Barbell Wide Grip Row
- Barbell Close Grip Row
- Dumbbell Wide Grip Row
- Dumbbell Close Grip Row
- One-Arm Dumbbell Row
- Lat Pulldown (to the front)
- Lat Pulldown (to the back)
- Bodyweight Pull-up (different grip variations)

- Bodyweight Chin-up (different grip variations)
- Assisted Pull-up (different grip variations)
- Assisted Chin-up (different grip variations)
- Weighted Pull-up (different grip variations)
- Weighted Chin-up (different grip variations)
- Barbell Deadlift
- Dumbbell Deadlift
- Smith Machine Deadlift
- Barbell Stiff-leg Deadlift
- Dumbbell Stiff-leg Deadlift
- Smith Machine Stiff-leg Deadlift
- Straight Arm Cable Pulldown
- Reverse Fly
- Barbell Pullover
- Dumbbell Pullover
- Machine Pullover
- Barbell Upright Row
- EZ-Curl Bar Upright Row
- Dumbbell Upright Row
- T-bar Row
- Smith Machine Wide Grip Row
- Smith Machine Close Grip Row
- Barbell Shrug
- Dumbbell Shrug
- Smith Machine Shrug

Samples of Back Workouts

Workout #1

Wide Grip Pulldowns 3x8-12
Close Grip Pulldowns 3x8-12
Wide Grip Barbell Rows 3x8-12
Close Grip Dumbbell Rows 3x8-12
Barbell Shrugs 3x8-12

Workout #2

Wide Grip Pulldowns 3x8-12
Neutral Grip Pulldowns 3x8-12
Wide Grip Dumbbell Row 3x8-12
T-bar Rows 3x8-12
Dumbbell Shrugs 3x8-12

Workout #3

Wide Grip Pull-up 3x8-12
Close Grip Chin-up3x8-12
Smith Machine Wide Grip Row 3x8-12
Smith Machine Close Grip Row 3x8-12
Smith Machine Shrugs 3x8-12

Workout #4

Close Grip Pull-up 3x8-12
Wide Grip Chin-up 3x8-12
Straight Arm Cable Pullover 3x8-12
T-bar Row 3x8-12
Barbell Shrugs 3x8-12

<u>Workout #5</u>

Assisted Pull-up 3x8-12
Assisted Chin-up 3x8-12
Barbell Stiff-leg Deadlift 3x8-12
Barbell Upright Row 3x8-12
Dumbbell Pullover 3x8-12

The Biceps

Anatomy of the Biceps

Biceps Brachii:

The biceps brachii is given the name "biceps" (plural) because it has two heads, and brachii comes from the Latin word for arm.

The short head of the biceps attaches to the coracoid process of the scapula. The tendon of the long head passes into the joint capsule at the head of the humerus and attaches on the scapula at the supraglenoid tubercle.

Distally, the biceps attaches to the radial tuberosity. The biceps also connect with the fascia of the medial side of the arm, at the bicipital aponeurosis.

Brachialis:

It arises from the distal, anterior half of the humerus and the intermuscular septa. It inserts into the coronoid process and tuberosity of the ulna over the elbow joint.

Pronator Teres:

It arises from the distal end of the medial humerus and the medial part of the ulna. From there it inserts into the lateral side of the radius.

Different Parts of the Biceps

The biceps brachii is a muscle on the upper arm that acts to flex the elbow. Since the biceps is attached to the radial tuberosity, this bone can rotate which allows the biceps to also supinate the forearm.

The brachialis is the main flexor of the forearm.

The job of the pronator teres is to pronate at the forearm and to also flex the forearm at the elbow.

Different Biceps Exercises

- Barbell Biceps Curl
- Dumbbell Biceps Curl
- Straight Bar Cable Machine Biceps Curl
- EZ Bar Cable Machine Close Grip Biceps Curl
- EZ Bar Cable Machine Wide Grip Biceps Curl
- Overhead Cable Machine Curl
- Dumbbell Hammer Curl
- Cable Machine Hammer Curl
- EZ Bar Close Grip Biceps Curl

- EZ Bar Wide Grip Biceps Curl
- Cable Machine Preacher Curl
- Straight Bar Preacher Curl
- EZ Bar Close Grip Preacher Curl
- EZ Bar Wide Grip Preacher Curl
- Dumbbell Preacher Curl
- Cable Machine Preacher Hammer Curl
- Incline Dumbbell Biceps Curl
- Dumbbell Concentration Curl
- Reverse Barbell Curl
- Barbell 21's

Samples of Biceps Workouts

Workout #1

Barbell Curls 3x8-12
Incline Dumbbell Curls 3x8-12
Preacher Curls 3x8-12

Workout #2

Dumbbell Curls 3x8-12
Reverse Barbell Curls 3x8-12
Barbell 21's 3x8-12

Workout #3

EZ Bar Close Grip Curls 3x8-12
EZ Bar Wide Grip Curls 3x8-12

Cable Rope Hammer Curls 3x8-12

Workout #4

Straight Bar Cable Machine Biceps Curls 3x8-12
Incline Dumbbell Curls 3x8-12
Dumbbell Hammer Curls 3x8-12

Workout #5

Dumbbell Biceps Curl 3x8-12
Straight Bar Cable Machine Biceps Curl 3x8-12
Barbell 21's 3x8-12

Workout #6

EZ Bar Cable Machine Close Grip Biceps Curls 3x8-12
EZ Bar Cable Machine Wide Grip Biceps Curls 3x8-12
Dumbbell Preacher Curls 3x8-12

Workout #7

Barbell Curls 3x8-12
Seated Dumbbell Curls 3x8-12
Dumbbell Hammer Curls 3x8-12

Workout #8

Barbell Curls 3x8-12

Barbell Reverse Curls 3x8-12
Barbell Preacher Curls 3x8-12

There are many different ways that you can stimulate the biceps, direct/indirect and both. You can use just about anything in the gym to stimulate the muscle (barbell, dumbbell, cables, tubing, bodyweight). You can use several different techniques to stimulate the muscle as well: negatives, super-sets, rest-pause, 21's, and super slow training just to name a few. However, the best single exercise to put some serious mass on your biceps is the straight barbell curl. This should be utilized at the beginning of your workout when you have the most energy.

The Calf

Anatomy of the Calf

Gastrocnemius:

The gastrocnemius is also called the calf muscle. The muscle itself is one that is visible on the body (meaning it doesn't lie underneath any other muscles and therefore is visible to the eye). The gastrocnemius attaches to the heel (at the Achilles Tendon) and originates on the femur (behind the knee). The calf muscle has two heads (the medial and lateral heads).

Soleus:

Unlike the gastrocnemius, this is one of those muscles that I mentioned above that are not visible because it lies underneath another muscle. It is for this reason that the muscle isn't very well known among those just starting out. The medial head originates on the posterior tibia and the lateral head on the posterior fibula. These two heads unite and insert into the calcaneal tendon.

Plantaris:

The plantaris is a very small muscle. The long tendon of the plantaris passes between the gastrocnemius and soleus and inserts into the calcaneus. It originates at the lateral epicondyle of the femur, just above the origin of the lateral head of the gastrocnemius.

Different Parts of the Calf

Gastrocnemius:

The function of this muscle is plantar flexion (elevating the heel). Without this muscle, it would be very hard to walk normally since you would not be able to push off the ball of your foot.

Soleus:

The function of this muscle is basically the same as the gastrocnemius in that its job is to raise the heel.

The only real difference between the two is that the soleus comes into play when the knee is bent (for example during seated calf raises).

Plantaris:

This is a very weak muscle but does help aid in raising the heel (plantar flexion).

Different Calf Exercises

- Standing Barbell Calf Raises
- Seated Barbell Calf Raises
- Smith Machine Standing Calf Raises
- Smith Machine Reverse Standing Calf Raises
- Smith Machine Seated Calf Raises
- Standing Dumbbell Calf Raises
- Seated Dumbbell Calf Raises
- Standing Cable Calf Raises
- Donkey Calf Raises
- Calf Press on Leg Press Machine
- Single-Leg Dumbbell Calf Raises
- Machine Standing Calf Raises
- Machine Seated Calf Raises

Samples of Calf Workouts

It is important to know that for many people the calf responds better to higher rep sets. See what works for you, but for most people, you will need to be doing at least 15 reps per set. The reason behind this is because the calf is a muscle you use regularly. Every time you take a step, your calf muscles are engaged. For this reason, they have built up endurance and to really activate the muscle you will need to apply heavy resistance with a lot of reps.

You want to concentrate on really feeling the calf contracting during the set and get a good stretch at the bottom of the movement and a hard contraction at the top.

Do not bounce during the movement. You want to make sure that during both the concentric and eccentric part of the movement is nice and slow and controlled.

Workout #1

Standing Barbell Calf Raises 4x15
Seated Barbell Calf Raises 4x15
Donkey Calf Raises 4x15

Workout #2

Standing Barbell Calf Raises 4x15
Standing One-Leg Dumbbell Calf Raises 4x15
Seated Dumbbell Calf Raises 4x15

Workout #3

Smith Machine Standing Calf Raises 4x15
Standing One-Leg Calf Raises 4x15
Donkey Calf Raises 4x15

Workout #4

Calf Press on Leg Press Machine 4x15
Machine Standing Calf Raises 4x15
Machine Seated Calf Raises 4x15

Workout #5

Calf Press on Leg Press Machine 4x15
Standing Barbell Calf Raises 4x15
Machine Seated Calf Raises 4x15

Workout #6 (Smith Machine)

Smith Machine Reverse Standing Calf Raises
4x15
Smith Machine Standing Calf Raises 4x15
Smith Machine Seated Calf Raises 4x15

Workout #7 (Bodyweight)

Standing Bodyweight Calf Raises 6x15
Standing One-Leg Bodyweight Calf Raises 6x15

The Chest

Anatomy of the Chest

The chest is made up of two muscles: the pectoralis major and the pectoralis minor.

The pecs are found attached to the humerus of the arm, right near where the shoulder joint is. They then run across the front of the body and originate on the breastbone. The pectoralis major is attached to the front of the body on the rib cage. The pectoralis minor is found underneath the pectoralis major. It originates on the ribs and attaches up to the scapula, specifically at the coracoid process.

The pectoralis major brings the humerus across the body while the pectoralis minor moves the shoulders forward. Together, you get the bench press pushing movement.

Like I mentioned earlier, once you understand how everything works it makes it much easier to visualize the muscle fibers contracting during each set. When you have a good mind-muscle connection you get more out of each rep. Too many people try to load on a weight that they can't handle and end up using more accessory muscles rather than the chest alone. That's fine if you are trying to impress someone, but in terms of results, it's not efficient.

Different Parts of the Chest

When hitting the chest, you have 3 different areas that you want to hit hard with compound movements. You have the upper chest, mid-chest, and lower chest.

The upper chest is something that some people forget about. The best exercise for hitting the upper chest is incline barbell presses. For this, you want to have the bench on an incline where you can specifically feel it working your upper chest. Different people feel the exercise at different angles (45 degrees works for most people)—but the best thing to do is try different angles to see what works for you.

If you feel the exercise more towards the middle of your chest, then you have the angle too low and it will feel more like a flat bench press. On the flip side, if you feel the exercise more in your shoulders, then you have the angle too high and you need to decrease the angle.

The mid-chest is hit with the famous exercise—the bench press. You see all the guys in the gym doing it during one of their workouts. An industry joke is that Monday is international chest day. Too many people are in the gym trying to impress everyone with how much they can bench, yet more than half of them are doing the exercise incorrectly in which they can cause serious injury to themselves.

The famous saying, "What do you bench?" is asked around the gym more than any other question—I cringe at the sound of it. Not because I don't care what they bench, but because I know that person is one of the many that I mentioned above that are probably executing the exercise incorrectly. So, let me say it once and get it over with… It's not how much weight you can lift, leave your ego at the door—concentrate on feeling the weight and using the correct form. Another exercise that involves no weights that hits the mid-chest is the pushup. These are great for if you can't get to the gym or you want to pump up a little bit.

The lower chest I believe is the most neglected portion of the chest. When you look at the best chests in fitness you notice from top to bottom the chest is fully developed and full. If someone neglects the lower portion of their chest you will notice fullness in the upper half but below mid-chest, they will be flat and without the roundness at the bottom portion. Doing decline presses as well as dips can help develop the lower chest.

Different Chest Exercises

- Flat Barbell Bench Press
- Flat Dumbbell Bench Press
- Incline Barbell Bench Press
- Incline Dumbbell Bench Press
- Decline Barbell Bench Press
- Decline Dumbbell Bench Press
- Flat Bench Dumbbell Flys
- Incline Bench Dumbbell Flys
- Decline Bench Dumbbell Flys
- Flat Dumbbell Press on the Stability Ball
- Flat Dumbbell Fly on the Stability Ball
- Flat Cable Machine Fly on the Stability Ball
- Smith Machine Flat Bench Press
- Smith Machine Incline Bench Press
- Smith Machine Decline Bench Press
- Machine Fly
- Pec Deck
- Cable Machine Flat Bench Fly
- Cable Machine Incline Bench Fly
- Cable Machine Decline Bench Fly
- Bodyweight Pushups (different hand positions available)
- Weighted Pushups (different hand positions available)
- Bodyweight Incline Pushups on the Stability Ball (different hand positions available)
- Bodyweight Dips
- Assisted Dips
- Weighted Dips
- Pullovers

Samples of Chest Workouts

Workout #1

Incline Barbell Bench Press 3x8-12
Flat Barbell Bench Press 3x8-12
Decline Barbell Bench Press 3x8-12
Incline Bench Dumbbell Fly 3x15
Flat Bench Dumbbell Fly 3x15

Workout #2

Incline Dumbbell Press 3x8-12
Flat Dumbbell Press 3x8-12
Decline Dumbbell Press 3x8-12
Incline Cable Fly 3x15
Flat Cable Fly 3x15

Workout #3

Incline Dumbbell Press 3x8-12
Flat Barbell Bench Press 3x8-12
Dips 3x8-12
Incline Dumbbell Fly 3x15
Machine Fly 3x15

Workout #4 (bodyweight workout)

Bodyweight Incline Pushup on Stability Ball 5x8-12
Bodyweight Pushup 5x8-12

Bodyweight Dips 5x8-12

<u>Workout #5 (Smith Machine workout)</u>

Smith Machine Incline Bench Press 5x8-12
Smith Machine Flat Bench Press 5x8-12
Smith Machine Decline Bench Press 5x8-12

The Hamstrings

Anatomy of the Hamstrings

The hamstrings are made up of three muscles. Those three muscles are the biceps femoris, semimembranosus, and the semitendinosus.

All three of these muscles originate on the pelvic bone under the glutes and then insert on the tibia.

The biceps femoris, semimembranosus, and the semitendinosus are all used for flexing the knee as well as hip extension. For those of you who aren't familiar with that terminology, think of knee flexion as a leg curl—where you are taking your foot and moving it towards your glutes in one fluid motion. An example of hip extension is where you are moving your leg to the rear. You can think of the movement like a stiff-leg deadlift.

Different Parts of the Hamstrings

Biceps Femoris

The biceps femoris is a muscle that like its name says (bi-), therefore having two heads. There is a long as well as a short head to the muscle.

The long head of the muscle starts at the lower and inner impression of the tuberosity of the ischium on the backside. For those who are not sure where that is located, think of it attaching to the back of the hip bone. It then travels down and inserts on the lateral condyle of the tibia.

The short head of the muscle starts between the adductor magnus and the vastus lateralis and extends up as high as the insertion of the glute muscles. The adductor magnus originates on the lower portion of the ischial tuberosity and is inserted onto the tubercle below the medial condyle on the tibia. The adductor magnus is responsible for hip extension.

Semimembranosus

The semimembranosus is located at on the medial side on the back of the thigh. The muscle originates on the hip, specifically the tuberosity of the ischium. From there it travels down and inserts onto the medial condyle of the tibia on the lower leg.

Semitendinosus

The semitendinosus is located at the medial and posterior area of the thigh and originates from the same place as the semimembranosus (the tuberosity of the ischium found on the hip). From there it travels down and inserts onto the upper part of the medial surface of the tibia.

Different Hamstring Exercises

- Seated Leg Curls
- Lying Leg Curls
- Standing Leg Curls
- Lying Bodyweight Flutter Kicks
- Stability Ball Flutter Kicks
- Barbell Stiff-Leg Deadlifts
- Dumbbell Stiff-Leg Deadlifts
- Dumbbell Lunges
- Barbell Lunges
- Smith Machine Stiff-Leg Deadlifts
- Squats
- Glute-Ham Raises
- Barbell Good Mornings

Samples of Hamstring Workouts

Workout #1

Squats 3x8-12
Dumbbell Lunges 3x8-12
Smith Machine Stiff-Leg Deadlifts 3x8-12
Glute-Ham Raises 3x8-12

Workout #2

Lying Leg Curls 3x8-12
Barbell Lunges 3x8-12
Dumbbell Stiff-Leg Deadlifts 3x8-12
Barbell Good Mornings 3x8-12

Workout #3

Standing Leg Curls 3x8-12
Barbell Stiff-Leg Deadlift 3x8-12
Dumbbell Lunges 3x8-12
Stability Ball Flutter Kicks 3x8-12

Workout #4

Squats 3x8-12
Barbell Stiff-Leg Deadlift 3x8-12
Glute-Ham Raise 3x8-12
Lying Bodyweight Flutter Kicks 3x8-12

Workout #5

Barbell Stiff-Leg Deadlift 3x8-12
Barbell Lunges 3x8-12
Lying Leg Curls 3x8-12
Glute-Ham Raises 3x8-12

Workout #6

Seated Leg Curls 3x8-12
Dumbbell Stiff-Leg Deadlift 3x8-12
Dumbbell Lunges 3x8-12
Barbell Good Mornings 3x8-12

The Neck

Anatomy of the Neck

The neck is made up of several muscles—ranging from flexors and extensors, to rotators and lateral flexors. Flexors are responsible for moving your chin towards your chest. Extensors are responsible for moving your head backward so you can look up. Rotators allow you to look from side to side. Lateral flexors are responsible for moving your ear towards your shoulder.

Different Parts of the Neck

Flexors
- Longus Colli
- Longus Capitis
- Infrahyoids

Extensors
- Splenius Capitis
- Semispinalis Capitis
- Suboccipitals
- Trapezius

Rotators
- Splenius Capitis
- Sternocleidomastoid
- Levator Scapula

- Suboccipitals

<u>Lateral Flexors</u>
- Scalenes

<u>Where are the neck muscles located?</u>

Longus Colli- The longus colli is found at the front of the spine. There are three portions of the longus colli—superior oblique, inferior oblique, and a vertical. The longus colli can be found between the atlas and the third thoracic vertebra on the anterior surface of the vertebral column.

Longus Capitis- The longus capitis is thick at the top and narrows as it descends. It is found on the anterior tubercles of the transverse processes of the 3rd, 4th, 5th, 6th cervical vertebrae. The longus capitis then inserts on the inferior surface of the basilar part of the occipital bone.

Infrahyoids- The infrahyoids are depressor muscles of the larynx.

Splenius Capitis- The splenius capitis is found from the spinous processes of the upper three or four thoracic vertebrae and also from the ligamentum nuchae from the 7th cervical vertebra. It then travels upward and is inserted into the mastoid process and also into the superior nuchal line.

Semispinalis Capitis- The semispinalis capitis is found at the back of the neck at the 7th cervical vertebrae and from the three cervical vertebrae above on the articular processes. It inserts between the superior and inferior nuchal lines of the occipital bone.

Suboccipitals- The suboccipitals are found at the first two cervical vertebrae and insert on the transverse process of the first cervical vertebrae and also on the occipital bone.

Trapezius- The trapezius is the large muscle of the upper back. It is found on the medial part of the superior nuchal line, ligament nuchae, spinous processes, and supraspinous ligaments to T12 and is inserted on the lower to medial acromion and superior spine of the scapula to the deltoid tubercle.

Sternocleidomastoid- The sternocleidomastoid is found on the anterior and superior manubrium and superior medial third of the clavicle and inserts on the lateral aspect of the mastoid process and the anterior half of the superior nuchal line.

Levator Scapula- The levator scapula is found on the posterior tubercles of the transverse processes of C1-4 and is inserted on the upper part of the medial border of the scapula.

Scalenes- The scalenes are found from the lateral processes of the cervical vertebrae of C3 to C7 and insert onto the 1st and 2nd ribs. They are a grouping of three pairs of muscles—the anterior scalene, middle scalene, and the posterior scalene.

Different Neck/Trap Exercises

- Isometric Neck Exercise - Front and Back
- Isometric Neck Exercise - Sides
- Lying Face-Down Plate Neck Resistance
- Lying Face-Up Plate Neck Resistance
- Seated Head Harness Neck Resistance
- Standing Head Harness Neck Resistance
- Barbell Shrugs
- Smith Machine Shrugs
- Dumbbell Shrugs
- Cable Shrugs
- Barbell Upright Rows
- Dumbbell Upright Rows
- Cable Upright Rows

Samples of Neck/Trap Workouts

Workout #1

Isometric Neck Exercise (Front) 3x8-12
Isometric Neck Exercise (Back) 3x8-12
Isometric Neck Exercise (Sides) 3x8-12
Barbell Shrugs 3x8-12

Workout #2

Face-Up Plate Resistance 3x8-12
Face-Down Plate Resistance 3x8-12
Isometric Neck Exercise (Sides) 3x8-12
Dumbbell Shrugs 3x8-12

Workout #3

Seated Head Harness Neck Resistance (Front)
3x8-12
Seated Head Harness Neck Resistance (Back)
3x8-12
Isometric Neck Exercise (Sides) 3x8-12
Smith Machine Shrugs 3x8-12

Workout #4

Isometric Neck Exercise (Front) 3x8-12
Isometric Neck Exercise (Back) 3x8-12
Isometric Neck Exercise (Sides) 3x8-12
Barbell Upright Row 3x8-12

Workout #5

Seated Head Harness Neck Resistance (Front)
3x8-12

Seated Head Harness Neck Resistance (Back)
3x8-12
Isometric Neck Exercise (Sides) 3x8-12
Dumbbell Upright Rows 3x8-12

<u>Workout #6</u>

Face-Up Plate Resistance 3x8-12
Face-Down Plate Resistance 3x8-12
Isometric Neck Exercise (Sides) 3x8-12
Cable Upright Rows 3x8-12

The Quadriceps

Anatomy of the Quadriceps

The quads are made up of 4 muscles (vastus medialis, vastus intermedius, vastus lateralis, rectus femoris). These 4 muscles are found on the front of the thigh. They originate at the top of the femur (largest bone in the leg) and attach down on the tibia.

The rectus femoris, however, is a little different in that it goes across the hip joint and originates on the pelvis itself. It is the combination of low body fat and massive muscle that gives you that nice cut teardrop look that is shown on the bodybuilding stage. Without low body fat, your hard work will be distorted by fat and water.

The purpose of the quads is to straighten and extend the knee (think about a leg extension). The purpose of the rectus femoris is to extend the knee, but it is also a hip flexor.

Different Parts of the Quadriceps

Let's start off by explaining and defining the quadriceps. The term "quad" means four. Therefore, the quadriceps are made up of 4 distinct muscles as mentioned above.

The front of the quad is made up of the rectus femoris. Directly underneath the rectus femoris is the vastus intermedius. Then on either side of both, you will find muscles that run parallel. These are the vastus medialis (on the inside of the leg) and the vastus lateralis (on the outside of the leg).

Different Quad Exercises

- Barbell Back Squats
- Barbell Front Squats
- Barbell Hack Squats
- Bodyweight Sissy Squat
- Weighted Sissy Squat
- Barbell Side Split Squats
- Barbell Single-Leg Squat
- Dumbbell Squats
- Bodyweight Jump Squat
- Jefferson Squat
- Zecher Squat
- Smith Machine Squat
- Smith Machine One-Leg Squat
- Leg Extensions
- Barbell Step-Ups
- Dumbbell Step-Ups
- Close-Stance Leg Press
- Wide-Stance Leg Press
- Barbell Lunges
- Dumbbell Lunges

- Walking Barbell Lunges
- Walking Dumbbell Lunges
- Barbell Deadlifts
- Dumbbell Deadlifts
- Smith Machine Deadlift
- Cable Hip Abduction
- Cable Hip Adduction
- Machine Hip Abduction
- Machine Hip Adduction

Samples of Quad Workouts

Workout #1

Barbell Squats 3x8-12
Leg Press 3x8-12
Walking Lunges 3x8-12
Leg Extension 3x8-12

Workout #2

Barbell Squat 3x8-12
Barbell Front Squat 3x8-12
Barbell Deadlift 3x8-12
Barbell Step-Ups 3x8-12

Workout #3

Smith Machine Squat 3x8-12
Dumbbell Deadlift 3x8-12
Close-Stance Leg Press 3x8-12

Walking Dumbbell Lunges 3x8-12

Workout #4

Jefferson Squat 3x8-12
Smith Machine Deadlift 3x8-12
Wide-Stance Leg Press 3x8-12
Leg Extension 3x8-12

Workout #5

One-Leg Squat 3x8-12 (each leg)
Bodyweight Jump Squat 3x8-12
Hip Abduction 3x8-12
Hip Adduction 3x8-12

The Shoulder

Anatomy of the Shoulder

The shoulder is the most movable joint in the body and because of this is very unstable. The shoulder itself is a ball and socket joint. The ball of the shoulder is the head of the humerus. The socket portion of the shoulder is called the glenoid (where arthritis in the shoulder forms). On top of the ball and socket is a process called the acromion (where bone spurs can form). Next to the acromion is the acromioclavicular joint, also called the AC Joint (this is a common place for shoulder separations). This ball and socket joint allows for the most range of motion out of all the joints in the body.

The roundness that you see at your shoulder is actually made up of 3 separate muscles or "heads". These heads are the anterior, middle, and posterior deltoid muscles. The deltoid is a pinnate muscle, which is where the muscle with fascicles attaches obliquely to its tendon. This allows better force production and stabilization, but you lose some flexibility.

Different Parts of the Shoulder

Anterior Deltoid

The anterior deltoid originates on the clavicle and inserts onto the deltoid tuberosity of the humerus. The main job of the anterior deltoid is shoulder abduction when the shoulder is externally rotated, but it also assists with transverse flexion but it is not a strong movement for this part of the deltoid.

Middle Deltoid

The middle deltoid originates on the acromion of the shoulder blade and inserts onto the deltoid tuberosity of the humerus. The purpose of the middle deltoid is shoulder abduction when the shoulder is internally rotated and also assists in shoulder transverse abduction.

Posterior Deltoid

The posterior deltoid originates on the spine of the scapula and inserts onto the deltoid tuberosity of the humerus. The posterior deltoid aids in shoulder extension, external rotation, transverse abduction and also transverse extension.

Rotator Cuff

Another key component of the shoulder is the rotator cuff. This is a place for common injuries to take place due to overuse or underuse (lack of use decreases strength and tears when overworked). The rotator cuff is made up of four muscles; the teres minor, infraspinatus, supraspinatus, and subscapularis. These four muscles are what aid in all overhead and rotational movements at the shoulder.

Different Shoulder Exercises

- Barbell Front Raises
- Dumbbell Front Raises
- Cable Front Raises
- Dumbbell Lateral Raises
- Cable Lateral Raises
- Bent-Over Lateral Raises
- Cable Rear Delt Reverse Fly
- Arnold Presses
- Military Presses
- Barbell Shoulder Press
- Dumbbell Shoulder Press
- Barbell Upright Rows
- Dumbbell Upright Rows
- Cable Upright Rows

Samples of Shoulder Workouts

Workout #1

Dumbbell Front Raises 3x8-12
Dumbbell Side Lateral Raises 3x8-12
Bent-Over Lateral Raises 3x8-12

Dumbbell Shoulder Press 3x8-12

Workout #2

Barbell Front Raises 3x8-12
Cable Lateral Raises 3x8-12
Cable Rear Delt Reverse Fly 3x8-12
Military Presses 3x8-12

Workout #3

Cable Front Raises 3x8-12
Dumbbell Side Lateral Raises 3x8-12
Bent-Over Lateral Raises 3x8-12
Arnold Presses 3x8-12

Workout #4

Dumbbell Front Raises 3x8-12
Cable Lateral Raises 3x8-12
Cable Rear Delt Reverse Fly 3x8-12
Barbell Shoulder Press 3x8-12

Workout #5

Cable Front Raises 3x8-12
Cable Side Lateral Raises 3x8-12
Cable Rear Delt Reverse Fly 3x8-12
Arnold Presses 3x8-12

The Triceps

Anatomy of the Triceps

The triceps brachii (better known as the triceps) has three heads—lateral, medial, long. All three heads of the triceps are connected to the humerus and scapula bones. The muscle then travels down the arm and is connected on to the ulna of the forearm.

Lateral Head:
The lateral head of the triceps is found on the outer side of the humerus. This section of the triceps is what makes up the horseshoe shape of the triceps when flexed.

Medial Head:
The medial head of the triceps is found in the middle of the back portion of the upper arm.

Long Head:
The long head of the triceps is the largest part of the triceps and is found running down the back of the arm along the body.

Different Parts of the Triceps

The primary function of all parts of the triceps is to straighten the arm by extending at the elbow.

Picture this movement as a triceps pushdown using a cable machine where your arm is bent at the elbow and as you push down using your triceps, your arm becomes straight at the bottom of the movement.

The long head of the triceps has one main function and that is to adduct the arm down to the body.

Different Triceps Exercises

- Reverse-Grip Bench Presses
- Smith Machine Reverse-Grip Bench Press
- Close-Grip Bench Press
- Smith Machine Close-Grip Bench Press
- Dumbbell Tate Press
- Dips Between Benches
- Weighted Dips Between Benches
- Machine Dips
- Parallel Bar Dips
- Weighted Parallel Bar Dips
- Assisted Dip Machine
- Push-Ups (hands closer than shoulder-width)
- One-Arm Dumbbell Triceps Extensions
- Two-Dumbbell Triceps Extensions
- Cable Reverse Pushdowns
- Cable One-Arm Pushdowns
- Cable Straight-Bar Pushdowns

- Cable Rope Pushdowns
- Cable V-Bar Pushdowns
- One-Arm Rope Pushdowns
- Dumbbell Triceps Kickbacks
- One-Arm Cable Triceps Kickbacks
- Standing Barbell Triceps Extensions
- One-Dumbbell Triceps Extensions
- Lying Barbell Triceps Extensions
- Incline Barbell Triceps Extensions
- Lying Cable Triceps Extensions
- Overhead Cable Triceps Extensions
- Overhead One-Arm Cable Triceps Extensions
- Skull Crushers
- Decline Skull Crushers
- JM Press

Samples of Triceps Workouts

Workout #1

Close-Grip Bench Press 4x8-12
Cable Straight Bar Pushdowns 4x8-12
Dumbbell Triceps Kickbacks 4x8-12

Workout #2

Barbell Reverse-Grip Bench Press 4x8-12
Cable V-Bar Pushdowns 4x8-12
Dumbbell Tate Press 4x8-12

Workout #3

Weighted Dips 4-8-12
Skull Crushers 4x8-12
Overhead Cable Triceps Extensions 4x8-12

Workout #4

JM Presses 4x8-12
Cable Rope Pushdowns 4x8-12
Dumbbell Kickbacks 4x8-12

Workout #5

Decline Skull Crushers 4x8-12
Cable Straight-Bar Reverse Pushdowns 4x8-12
Overhead One-Arm Cable Triceps Extensions
4x8-12

Workout #6

Standing Barbell Triceps Extensions 4x8-12
One-Arm Rope Pushdowns 4x8-12
Assisted Dip Machine 4x8-12

Workout #7

Standing Barbell Triceps Extensions 4x8-12
One-Dumbbell Triceps Extensions 4x8-12
Push-Ups (hands closer than shoulder-width)
4x8-12

Workout #8

Incline Barbell Triceps Extensions 4x8-12
Lying Cable Triceps Extensions 4x8-12
Machine Dips 4x8-12

How to Set Yourself Up for Success

- Goal Setting
- Choosing a Gym
- Picking a Training Partner
- Working Out with a Significant Other Who Hates Exercising
- Workouts While Traveling
- Eating Smart While Traveling
- Holiday Motivation

Goal Setting

What is a goal and why do we need them?

According to Dictionary.com, the definition of a goal is "the result or achievement toward which effort is directed; aim; end."

Now that we know the definition of a goal, let's break things down a bit.

A goal, especially in fitness, is something that you need to strive and work for. It is not something that can be handed to you and it is not something that will come easily. There will be many bumps in the road that you won't be prepared for and you will have to rise up to the occasion and get past those bumps.

Without goals in life, you have nothing to work towards. This can be something that you strive for in life as well as in the gym.

What types of goals work best?

The best types of goals that work best are those that are <u>specific and realistic</u>.

Goals need to be specific and to the point. For instance, if you were to say you want to get bigger, that is a goal but it is not specific. What does it mean? Do you want to get bigger by getting fat? I certainly hope not. You left out the specifics such as what you want to get bigger and how you plan on doing it. A better goal would be to say that you want to put on 1 inch of muscle mass to your chest and legs in a year's time. The reason this goal is better than the first is that it tells you exactly what you want to accomplish, with the details as well as a timeframe.

Details are important to goal setting because you want to make sure that you have something that you can measure over time. In the "better" example above, we are able to measure the progress of that goal. We can get out a tape measure and check the measurements of the chest and legs each week or month. Also, the "better" goal above is realistic. If the goal would have said that you want to put on 4 inches of muscle on the chest and legs, then that is something that cannot be accomplished in a year's time. Therefore, it is important to make the goal realistic because if you make it so hard and unrealistic, you will get frustrated and will more than likely give up.

Short and long-term goals

It is important to make both short and long-term goals. You want to have both so that you have an overall goal with a bunch of short-term goals that ensure that you are on the right path.

<u>Here is an example:</u>

Let's say you are looking to lose 45 pounds of fat in one year. Make that your overall long-term goal. If you left it at that, you have nothing to push for each week or month. Therefore, you need something to keep you on track and something that can be measured to ensure you are progressing toward your long-term goal. Your short-term goal would be each month you want to lose at least 4 pounds of fat. This is a realistic goal because you are able to safely lose 1-2 pounds a week which would equate to 4-8 pounds a month. This goal is also measurable by not only getting your body fat tested but also by hopping on the scale.

Utilizing both of these types of goals, you are able to make sure you are on track with your goal. Another positive aspect of these short-term goals is that you get positive reinforcement each month by measuring your results and seeing progress which will help you stick to your program.

<u>Write it down and check it often</u>

Writing down your goal is part of the mental process of committing to your goal. By writing it down, you are committing yourself to that goal. Think of it as written in stone. Under no circumstance can that goal not be attained.

If you are trying to lose weight, put your goal on the fridge or on the drawer that you keep your junk food in. That note that you wrote and placed on one of those spots (or both if need be) is a little reminder of your commitment to accomplish and stick with your weight loss goal.

On the other hand, if your goal is to put on lean muscle mass, then you can put a note basically anywhere you wish that would remind you about your commitment and keep you motivated and focused. Putting a note in your gym bag or on the pages of your workout journal should do the trick. Putting it on these places will remind you every time you open your gym bag or write down the reps for a given set on your journal that you have a purpose for going heavy and pushing your body to the limit.

The examples of where to put notes about your goal are just a couple off of the top of my head and are not the gospel of what should be done. Each of us is different and handle things differently. Find a place to put your goal and put it there and check it often—when you wake up, before you go to bed, whenever. You could even say your goal out loud each morning if you wish. If you continue to say your goal over and over again each day, you are basically training your mind to believe that you will achieve that goal (which is obviously what you want). The key here is to look at or say your goal as a reminder and motivation to keep pushing.

Everyone WANTS me to do this

NOOOOOOOOOOOOO! This is the wrong approach. Do not make a goal because everyone thinks or wants you to do something. You are simply setting yourself up for failure and might as well just quit now. The ONLY reason you should set a health or fitness goal is that YOU want to. No one else can fit into this equation.

If you don't want to do this for yourself, then what is your true motivation? To make someone else happy? Get out of here. To me, that is stupid and simply a waste of time and effort. Not only that but if you decide to go through with it and accomplish the goal, afterward there is no reason to continue because you already appeased whoever wanted you to reach that goal and have no reason to continue working hard or even maintain what you've accomplished.

<u>Don't expect to come out shooting like gang-busters</u>

The hardest thing to do after you make a goal is to get started. Going from a bad habit to a good habit isn't easy—I'm not going to lie to you. Take smoking for instance, if it was easy to quit then everyone would be quitting since they know it is bad for them and could kill them after continued use. Same goes for exercise. If being fit with a body fat under 10% with rock-hard abs and bulging muscles with striations all over were easy, then more than 60% of all American's wouldn't be overweight with more than 30% of those people being obese.

A lot of people complain that they don't have time to work out. That is a weak excuse. If it was a priority they would make time. When they decide to make a goal that involves exercise, some decide to get up early and hit the gym before work. Here comes problem number one. People are used to sleeping in each day until a certain time—now because of your goal, instead of waking up at 6 am you now have to wake up at 5 am. This for them might cause a problem. The alarm goes off, you hit the snooze because your body doesn't want to get out of bed. Too darn bad! This is where your dedication comes into play. It's about discipline. Force yourself out of your bed, put on your workout apparel and get it done.

Take your time and don't get frustrated. Too many people drop out and give up because they expect to see results and changes right away. For most people, physical changes due to exercise can take anywhere from weeks to months depending on the person's body. Your body wants to keep itself in homeostasis—which is where it wants to stay the same at a constant level. When trying to lose weight, your body wants to fight you and keep all the fat cells that it currently has because as you diet and lower your calories, your body thinks it's going into starvation mode and wants to hold on to every last bit of fat you have for self-preservation. Stick to the plan and the results will come.

<u>Roadblocks</u>

Like I mentioned earlier, nothing comes easy. If things in life were easy, we would be stress-free. However, this is not the case for many of us.

During our journey to reaching our goals, there will be times that we screw-up or come to a fork-in-the-road and don't know which way to go. These screw-ups are part of the learning process that will help you stay focused and dedicated to your goals. They will help teach your brain to overcome obstacles and to find ways to overcome roadblocks. It might take a couple of trial-and-errors until you finally get it right, but that is half the battle of reaching a goal.

If you never had a roadblock on your way to a goal, then maybe the goal was too easy for you.

The key here is, if you fall off the wagon you need to get back on track and find the path to success. Don't turn around and call it quits because it is too hard, buckle down and go for it. When you achieve your goal and look back on what you went through to get there, it makes it much more rewarding.

Measurement

By measuring your progress, you will get both positive and negative reinforcement from your results. If you are bulking or cutting, the tape measure and body fat calipers don't lie. Despite what you want your numbers to be, measurement devices don't care if you are on the right path or not. They give you the cold hard facts whether you like it or not.

I recommend putting the results of your measurements either down on paper or on your laptop/smartphone. That way you have a log/journal of your progress. If you notice that you fell off track a little after getting your measurements done, then you know you need to get back on track. If you wouldn't have gotten things checked, you would have never known if you were progressing or regressing.

Choosing a Gym

Let's face it, there are a million different gyms out there today and all of them are a little bit different. You have your Planet Fitness for the individuals who are afraid of being judged in a real gym, you have the Powerhouse Gym's for the powerlifters, and you have the Gold's for the bodybuilders, and so on and so forth (other people do work out in each of those places as well). Finding one that you feel comfortable with is the key. If you join a gym where you are uncomfortable or intimidated, you will more than likely quit and give up. Therefore, it is important to really feel at home with whatever gym you choose.

So think about what you want in a gym. Are you strictly there to lift weights? Do you want to take aerobics classes? Do you strictly want it for the cardio equipment? Do you want all of these things? As you can see there are many options you need to think about when deciding what gym would suit you best. You need to think about what type of workout you want to get and go from there.

Let's go over some basics of choosing a gym that fits YOU...

<u>Questions to ask while visiting a gym…</u>

- What are the hours of operation?
- When are the busiest times of the day?
- How much does the membership cost? Are than any option plans available?
- What do you have to do to cancel?
- What are the billing cycles or can you pay it all upfront?
- Is the staff certified?
- Is the gym equipped and staff trained for emergencies?
- How old is the equipment?
- How often is the equipment replaced?
- What equipment gets used the most?
- Are the class sizes limited?
- Are there any extra fees involved or are all the services included in the price?
- Does the gym have childcare? If so is it free or how much is it?
- Do you get shown how to use the equipment free or is it fee-based?
- Do they do any free body composition testing or similar?

Things to Consider:

<u>Location</u>

Is the location of the gym accessible to you? You want to find a gym where you don't have to travel very far and that you know you wouldn't mind driving to. If the gym is too far and cuts into too much time of your day, more than likely you aren't going to stick with it too long or not as often as you would like.

Find a place that is possibly close to where you work so right before or after work you can go there or during a lunch hour. Look to see if there is anything close to your house. That will enable you to go to the gym whenever you want and you don't have to worry about cutting into precious time during the day—especially good when you are looking for a quick workout or some cardio.

<u>Hours of Operation</u>

Do their hours jive with your schedule? Can you comfortably get in a workout and not be pushed for time? You want to make sure that if you are paying for a membership that your workout schedule is well within their hours of operation, if not then you will be wasting your money by not being able to fully utilize their facility and get a good workout. Your best choice would be a gym that is open 24-hours a day if possible. That would ensure you that no matter what time it is, you can go get in a workout.

Cost

This should really be at the top of your list. How much money will it cost you and will you get your money's worth? It's much easier to spend a little extra money on a membership with a gym that has top of the line equipment and that is more inspirational to be in rather than a warn down gym that looks like a cave with equipment that is falling apart or sitting there broken.

You also need to realize what time of the year you are purchasing a membership. Gyms tend to have better deals during the high times of the year such as around New Years and in September. If you can hold off getting a membership until these times you will surely end up saving some money in the long run.

Make sure you are paying for exactly what you want for that price. Don't get coaxed into adding on services that you aren't going to use or paying for things that don't interest you. Many gyms will nickel and dime you to death, watch out for salesmen who run down a list of extra options/services that you could add to your membership. At that point, you're going to feel like you're buying a car.

Another thing you want to watch out for are gyms that make you lock in with a long-term agreement. These places will lock you into your contract for 1-3 years and there is no way to get out without huge cancellation fees. Say down the road you don't like the gym anymore or something happens which makes you not want to go there anymore, if you are locked in you have no way of getting out of the contract and will be forced to pay out the remaining balance or a cancellation fee. Now you are stuck paying for a gym that you won't use or dreading every day you force yourself to go just so you aren't wasting your money.

Cleanliness

How clean is the facility? Are there staff members who wipe down the equipment daily? Do they make sure members wipe down their equipment after using it? Is there trash on the floor? Are the locker rooms a mess? These are all things to consider when purchasing a membership. If the place looks like a mess you need to evaluate if that is something you can put up with every visit. For most people, a trashy gym is a huge turn-off. If they can't take care of their facility, how do you expect them to take care of you?

Membership Privileges and Features

Do you get discounts on anything they sell once you are a member? Do you get to tan and use the pool for free or is there an extra charge? Do they have massage therapists? Is there a gym child-care to take your kid(s) to while you work out? Is there a juice/smoothie or snack bar? How much will you be paying for these things?

You need to find out what extra features come with the membership and what you have to pay extra for. See if there are any perks to joining their gym over another one in the area. Make sure you understand exactly what comes with your membership and what doesn't before you sign any papers. Also, try to negotiate with them or have them throw in a few extra perks, it never hurts to ask. If they really want your business, they tend to cave a little bit. Just don't be a jerk in your approach.

Equipment

The equipment that you use needs to be in good working condition with no problems with its usage. Look at the different styles and brands of equipment that they have and make sure that it is something you are interested in using. How is the free weight area or room? Make sure the dumbbells aren't broken or that there aren't dumbbells missing or that one of the pairs isn't missing. Make sure the grips on the barbells aren't worn down so bad that they are completely smooth and your grip will be compromised. Look around to see how the members are handling the equipment. Are they dropping the dumbbells on the floor? Are they banging the barbell off the rack or ground? Are they slamming the machine weights down when they are done with a set?

If you see any of these things, be wary about the gym and the equipment. Surely there are going to be some serious issues and damages to equipment when they are used like that. Especially look to see how the staff handles a situation like that. If they have good equipment, they will definitely make sure things like that don't happen. If no one seems to care from the staff, more than likely their equipment will be broken down sooner rather than later. And also look around and see how many pieces of equipment are currently broken. If there are a lot of broken-down machines, it shows they don't take care of them and service them to keep them in proper working condition.

<u>Clientele</u>

What types of people are working out at the gym? Do you see mainly men? Do you see mainly women? Is there a good split between the two? Make sure you feel comfortable working around the people you see at the gym. Some gyms are known for being more hardcore such as the powerlifting gyms and the bodybuilding gyms. If you feel intimidated or unsafe being around these types of people when working out, then keep searching for a place that you can call home. Remember, searching for the right gym is all about you, no one else.

Atmosphere

How is the atmosphere of the gym? Is it upbeat or is it bland? Find a gym that is inspirational and makes you want to work out. There is nothing worse than going to a gym to work out and feel like you are stuck in a dreary day. Find a gym that is bright and energizes you. Look around and see how the members are interacting. Are they friendly or are they snobs? Comfort level plays a huge part in motivating yourself to go to the gym for a grueling workout.

Maintenance

There is nothing more frustrating than going to the gym to hit a body part and seeing that a piece you always use is broken. How quickly is a piece of equipment fixed after being broken? Do you go tell someone that the equipment isn't working and then when you come back a week later it is still broken? Some pieces of equipment do take some time to fix depending on the parts they have to order, but how quickly are they to accommodate to the situation? If it takes a long time to fix a piece of equipment, that is a tale-tell sign that they are pinching money and will hold off as long as possible to replace something just so they don't have to spend any money.

<u>Always try out the gym before you purchase a membership!</u>

No matter what you see, always try out the gym before you purchase a membership. You will make a big mistake if you just walk in and buy a membership without looking around at other options as well as seeing how the gym you are looking at is operating.

You want to ask for a trial membership, or a guest pass or anything they have that will allow you to try out the gym for at least a couple days. Most places will give you a pass to try it out, however for those who don't the average price for a day pass is roughly around $10 a day. Even if they make you pay, it will be well worth it to see if you like it. A $10 investment is much better than spending $500 and hating every minute. You want to go to the gym at the same time that you would normally work out. This will allow you to see how busy it gets during the times you are going to be there.

<u>When you decide on a gym, ALWAYS read the fine print before you sign!</u>

By reading the agreement and the fine print, it makes you aware of the contract you are signing. This can include how you will be paying for the membership, the term of the contract, cancellation policy, and other pertinent information that you need to know.

When it comes down to it you really need to take all of the things mentioned above into consideration. If you don't like something about the gym, check out some other places. The fitness industry is really taking off and gyms are popping up almost everywhere. Make sure you understand what you want before looking and make a list of things you want to look for and ask before you go visiting gyms. When you are there don't be afraid to ask questions. If the salesman tries to avoid any of your questions or is dancing around the question without truly answering it for you, place a checkmark next to that gym and keep looking. When it comes down to it, a gym membership is an investment—an investment in your health.

Picking the Perfect Training Partner

Ever feel like you can't get through a tough workout because you have no one pushing you, or have you ever felt like you couldn't do that one extra rep because you're afraid of dropping the weight on yourself? Many people feel that way all the time. It doesn't have to be like that as long as you have someone reliable to work out with.

Picking a training partner should not be a difficult task. The great thing about a workout partner is, you don't need to have a partner who is the same sex, they don't have to be the same age, and they don't have to be the same weight as you. Motivation can come from anyone.

Here are some things that you want to look for in a training partner:

Reliability

You ultimately want to pick someone who is reliable and who is there to help and push you during your workout. You also want someone who shows up at the scheduled meeting time. When you say you want to work out at 12 pm, that doesn't mean 12:10 pm or 12:20 pm. They need to be prompt and ready to work out when you are scheduled to meet.

Your partner should also be someone who doesn't take long absences from the gym. You don't want a partner who is constantly taking a couple of weeks off from lifting because of a "busy schedule" or because of X, Y, and Z.

Trustworthy

Your training partner should be there to push you through those last few reps that you wouldn't normally get by yourself. They should be trustworthy so while pushing your limits they can be there in case you need assistance with a weight or to help you with some forced reps. You want to have 100% faith in them to be there in case you need assistance.

Motivation

This shouldn't come as a shocker but when choosing a training partner, you want someone who can motivate you. If you have someone tagging along who doesn't make a sound the whole workout you might as well just be working out by yourself. Your training partner should help you get pumped up and wants you to be able to push harder and harder each workout.

<u>Knowledge</u>

The person you are training with needs to be knowledgeable in order to spot you correctly and safely (for the sake of both of you). Your partner should have some background knowledge of training so he/she isn't holding you back (unless both of you are just starting out and getting the feel for things).

If both you and your training partner are knowledgeable, you will have no problem changing up workouts every couple weeks to shock the muscles into new growth. Keeping things fresh allows you to never become bored with your workouts or time in the gym. By having things fresh and exciting you are more willing to adhere to the program versus going through the motions week in and week out.

<u>Goals</u>

Most people feel that they need a training partner that shares the same goals. To a point this is incorrect. Someone who is bulking and someone who is cutting can be doing the same exercises (the weights might vary though). As long as you have a partner who is there and motivates you, what he or she is trying to accomplish shouldn't affect you and your workout. The whole point of a training partner is someone to work out with and to help both of you reach your personal goals as well as provide motivation and assistance throughout your workouts.

Age

The great thing about training with a partner is that you don't have to be the same age. Someone in their 40's can easily train with someone in their 20's. Now the weights might not be the same, but each will be able to push the other and assist them when needed. It's also common to see a father or mother working out with their children. This is a great way to get a child off on the right foot (and off the couch) even at an early age.

Gender

It's not uncommon to see a husband and wife or a boyfriend and girlfriend working out together. In fact, this is a great way to bond and enjoy something together which will benefit you both in the long run. Most women can give men a good spot as long as they know how to spot the exercise correctly. Now in the case where men go to complete failure is when it might get a little hairy when the opposite sex needs to save them from a 300+ pound bar crashing down on the guy's chest. However, in most cases, women are strong enough to help men through a few forced reps regardless of the weight. Then again, you also have the cases where women can out lift the men and the roles are reversed.

Working Out with a Significant Other Who Hates Exercising

Let's face it, not everyone is keen on exercise. Or are they? Personally, I think everyone enjoys exercise, they just need to find out what form suits their needs and interests.

Working out with a wife/husband or significant other can be hard sometimes. What interests you might not interest them. It's a constant battle back and forth. How do you find a happy medium or how do you even get them started exercising? Most people want to exercise but they come up with excuses why they don't. Follow these steps and with a little luck, you might have just found yourself a new workout partner for life.

1) Why do they have a negative image of exercise?

This is the first step of the process. You need to converse with them and figure out what is causing them to hate exercise. Whatever it might be, you need to understand their needs and work around them.

They need to understand that there is a workout for everyone with every type of need.

2) What are their goals?

What are their goals? Do they even have any? Maybe they feel that they are a little overweight and wouldn't mind dropping a couple of pounds or maybe they feel they are too skinny and would like to put on some lean muscle mass.

Whatever the case is, you need to write down their goals. From there you need to come up with a plan of attack. How will you get them to achieve their goals without hating every minute of it?

3) Set short and long-term goals

Take the goals that they mentioned and look at them. Make some short and long-term goals that both of you agree upon. This is key, you need to make them a part of this process and not just lay it all out for them. If they have involvement in the process they will feel more comfortable knowing that you aren't making them do anything they don't want to do.

You want to make sure that the goals you are setting are measurable. It is important to have measurable goals because if you can't measure the progress then how will anyone know if there is ever any progress at all? Without seeing progress on paper or through pictures, the individual will more than likely get frustrated and lose interest altogether. The goal here is to show them that what they are doing is getting them closer to their ultimate goal.

The purpose of short-term goals is so that they are constantly getting positive reinforcement by achieving small goals that help them reach their ultimate goal. This will keep them motivated and on track. If you only have one ultimate goal, you lose sight of that goal after a while because it's such a huge transition that it could take a fairly long amount of time to reach. Therefore, they have small stepping-stones to reach throughout the process that help them towards their ultimate goal.

Those short-term goals need to lead to a long-term goal. This can be something as simple as losing 50 pounds in 8 months. We call it a long-term goal because as it says, it is a goal that will take a long time to reach when compared to the short-term goals.

I do want to note, I mentioned that the goals need to be measurable, but you also want to make sure they are achievable. Don't come up with goals that are so hard to achieve that the person cannot achieve. This will only deter them from exercise.

The goals should also be specific. Something general doesn't tell you much and it is hard to make good goals that can be measured. For instance, if you said you want to lose weight, that is very general. A better goal would be to say that you want to lose 50 pounds in one full year. This example allows you to measure your progress and gives you a goal to strive for.

4) Start off slow

Start off slow—this isn't a race. If you go out shooting like gangbusters you will lose sight of your goal because you rushed into things and didn't take the time to understand what you are doing and what changes your body is going through due to training.

Start off with just a couple of exercises per body part and work your way from there. Start with only 15 minutes of cardio if that is all they can do and work your way up to 30-60 minutes as they are showing improvement.

Remember, the tortoise beat the hare. Slow and steady always comes out on top. You find runners who start off sprinting in a race normally finish towards the back of the pack because they didn't ease their way into it. Same goes for those who jump into exercise by doing tons of reps and sets along with long cardio sessions. Take it slow and as progress is made, re-evaluate the training protocol and make changes where need be.

5) Introduce new things

As they are progressing, add in new fun things. Change up the exercises and change what they are doing for cardio. Flavor is the spice of life. Keep things fresh and fun and they won't get bored. If you find them not enjoying a certain exercise or cardio session, then change it up. You don't need to stick to one specific protocol— in most cases, you will find people constantly changing their workouts because they either get bored with it or they don't like the way an exercise feels. This is normal so don't make them do anything they don't enjoy just like you wouldn't want someone making you do something you didn't enjoy.

6) Give support

You are both in this together, and if your significant other is the one who isn't fond of exercise, they are going to need a lot of support and positive reinforcement. With that being said, you are their lifeline. When things aren't going well for them and they want to give up, you need to be there to pick them back up and encourage them to keep pushing. Without you being there with them, they wouldn't have started exercising in the first place, so you are the only one there to help them through this new journey.

When they are doing great, let them know so. Tell them they are making great progress and you can really see a difference in the way they look and how they present themselves. If they aren't doing so well, don't put them down, simply give them some motivation (a little kick in the butt) to help them get back on track.

7) Reward them

Now I'm not saying to go out and buy them a new car or anything like that, but little gifts to reward them for accomplishing goals never hurt anyone. Maybe buy them a new pair of running shoes or a new pair of workout pants. Something that they could use during their workout is the best gift to get them. It reinforces the purpose of working out and that they are achieving their set goals. Rewards are positive reinforcements that go a long way when giving them to someone who originally never wanted to start working out in the first place.

8) Enjoy each other's company

The main thing is to have fun. Enjoy each other's company and be each other's support system. You are both in this together to not only improve your overall health but to look better too. Don't work out and never make eye contact or break a smile. Have some fun, laugh a little while working out. You don't have to be serious when you work out, joke around and make things fun for both of you.

The more you enjoy spending time working out together, the more likely you are to make sure that you have a time set each day to plan for your workout. But again, I can't stress it enough… have fun working out and make it enjoyable for everyone involved. This is about a lifestyle change, so make it something that you enjoy and something that you both can enjoy for a lifetime. Who knows, maybe your significant other will soon enough be the one bugging you to get up extra early to get a workout in. Oh, how the tables can turn…

Workouts While Traveling

Are you a road warrior? Tend to spend most of your day in a car and in hotels? Being a road warrior isn't easy, that's for sure. Are you finding that your workouts are falling to the wayside and that your diet is going down the toilet? It doesn't have to be that way; with a little planning, you will be able to still maintain or improve your health and physique even though you are constantly on the road where nothing is consistent.

This section will give you some ideas and tips on how to make your travels more health and fitness-oriented.

Hotel Gyms

Let's face it, hotel gyms aren't the best for those of us who are accustomed to working out in a "real" gym or health club. Hotel gyms are normally small and only carry light dumbbells or possibly a couple of cable machine pieces that hit some of the major muscle groups. Normally the main pieces you will find in a hotel gym are cardio pieces. Most hotel gyms have treadmills, bikes, steppers, and even ellipticals. Other than that, the machines and free weights we are used to seeing are nowhere to be found. And that's okay.

Will this deter you from working out? I hope not! You just need to improvise. We all know that you are used to throwing around some serious weight, but obviously, right now you don't have a choice in the matter. You have to deal with what you got. With that being said, you need to change your workout around so that you can hit the body parts you want to hit with a good muscle-stimulating workout.

What does this mean? It means you have to go lighter and do more reps and sets. This isn't necessarily a bad thing. Think about it—you are used to doing heavy weights in the gym and that is primarily the only type of training you do weight resistance-wise. What have we all learned over the years of studying training protocols? You need to change things up to hit the muscle differently and force them into growing. It's all about stimulating the muscle and resting/feeding the muscle to recover and grow. So changing things up to a "light day" isn't the worst thing that can happen to you. In fact, it might help take your training and results to the next level.

Depending on what hotel you stay in, if the cardio equipment isn't your thing, some hotels have an indoor pool. This is not only a great place to relax and cool down after a workout, but it is also a great place to do cardio. Cardio in the pool can range from walking laps to swimming. If you are simply cooling down, I would recommend simply walking around in the pool. But if cardio is your mission, feel free to do some pool exercises like running in place and speed walking around the perimeter of the pool (depending on depth) to really bring the heart rate up.

The water in the pool gives you some resistance so it makes it a great all-around workout. Another incentive to use the pool for cardio is that it is very forgiving on the joints. The water prevents the heavy and constant pounding on the knees as compared to walking on concrete.

Gyms in the surrounding area

Obviously, if you are traveling, the majority of the time you will be staying in a hotel if you don't have friends in the surrounding area whose house you can crash at. If the hotel gym just doesn't do it for you, walk up to the front desk and ask them if there are any surrounding gyms or health clubs not too far from their location. Most of the time hotels and surrounding gyms partner up and exchange passes. If this is the case, they may be able to hook you up with a free day pass so you can use the local gym's facilities for free (free is good, right?).

You could always do a little research yourself, and beforehand you can surf the web and find gyms local to the hotel you will be staying at so you at least have an idea if one is available. I would say the MAJORITY of the time, there is always a gym local to a hotel, you just might need to ask or do some searching on the internet to find out where it is located.

If you don't mind the travel a little bit from the hotel and you need heavy weights, look for a local Gold's Gym, Powerhouse Gym, or another national chain as this will be your best bet in order to get in a workout that you are accustomed to doing when you are home and not traveling for business or pleasure.

If you plan on being in that area numerous times throughout the year, talk to a manager or sales consultant at the gym and see if they can hook you up with some type of deal where you can use the gym for so many visits for a certain price and in turn they will give you a punch card or something similar to use. They might even be cool with just giving you free day passes every time you are in town.

Another little trick that I have learned (I used to work in a gym so I know how it works) is if you go into a gym and mention that you are interested in joining the gym but you would like to try it out first, most of the time they will either let you try it out free for that day or they can give you a pass to allow you to use their facility for a couple of days. This will solve your workout problem while on the road.

The downside to this is that if you decide to go to their gym again in the future, they will have your name on file and will know you pulled one over on them the last time and will make you pay this go-around. But if you have no intention of going back to that gym, by all means, give my tip a try and see if you can score some free visits. What do you have to lose? The worst thing they could say is that they don't do free trials and they will make you pay a guest fee for the day. So give it a shot.

Portable gym equipment

For those of you who don't want to use the hotel gym and don't feel like finding a surrounding gym, I have just the thing for you! Resistance bands. I got them for when I am traveling on the road and can't find a gym in the area of the hotel. You can hit every muscle group with many different angles and exercises utilizing these bands. They are small enough that you can fit them in a small suitcase for use during travel or small enough to throw under the bed or in a drawer at home. I highly recommend them. They come in different resistances. Normally a light, moderate, heavy, and super-heavy is what you will find when shopping around.

<u>Food on the run</u>

This is extremely tough, probably the hardest things to do when you are constantly on the road traveling. Your main objective while on the road is obviously to make sales (assuming you're traveling on business)—with that being said you try and make as many stops as you can without too many interruptions. Most people end up going to a fast-food restaurant that is high in fat and calories simply because they can be in and out fairly quickly. I urge you to skip these types of places altogether if you can. But if you do decide to go, try and find a healthy option such as a grilled chicken sandwich. Lay off from all the sauces they put on, if it comes with lettuce and tomato, great, if not then just eat the grilled chicken breast and bun.

What I recommend to do is as soon as you get into a town or to start the day, head out a little early and hit up a grocery store. Get a gallon of water so you have it for all day long to sip on. You can also pick up some canned tuna or even some already prepared chicken breast that you can eat as meals or snacks throughout the day. Fruit and veggies are quick and easy to pick up at the store and eat in the car. Nuts are also a great option to carry around with you if you get hungry. It is very simple to plan out the day's meals, you just need to take the time to do it and get to the grocery store.

If you plan on carrying a lot of things that need to be kept cold, look into car refrigerators. They are small and compact and plug right into your cigarette lighter in your car. This makes it easy to carry water, protein shakes, and food that needs to be kept cool. In my opinion, they are worth the money in the long run if you travel frequently. They make planning meals quick and easy when all you need to do is open up the fridge right there in your car and grab a meal out of it.

If your company allows you to expense your meals and/or groceries while on the road, then you have it made. You can expense your grocery list and make sure you have the food you need throughout the day whether you prepare it or whether you have leftovers from a dinner out.

Stay hydrated

Like I mentioned above, the best thing to take on the road with you is water. Grab yourself a gallon of water and take it with you each day to sip on. It is very important (not just while on the road) to always stay hydrated. Water is very inexpensive and if you want you can fill up your gallon jug each day at the hotel if you don't feel like going out each day just to buy a gallon of water. Normally in the hotel gym, there is a water dispenser that you can easily hit up in the morning to refill your jug.

After a while, I do recommend throwing away the gallon jug and purchase a new one simply because of bacteria growth in the jug itself. I'd say use the same one no more than a couple of days unless you are washing it out after each use. The last thing you want to do when you are traveling is get sick. That makes traveling unbearable. Nothing like being stuck in a car all day while you are sick and needing to continually make stops throughout the day to take care of your "business".

Get plenty of rest

Sleep is a necessity not only when you are traveling, but for everyone in general. Most people don't get enough quality sleep each night. People stay up too late and wake up too early and never get their proper rest. This is common when on the road all day. Once you are done for the day and are in your hotel room, now you have to fill out all your paperwork or make your notes on your laptop about the day's events. This could mean your normal 8 or 9-hour day turns into a 10 to 12+ hour day. Add that up with the stress of being on the road and you could be on your way to getting sick due to not enough rest and the presence of high-stress levels.

Strive for at least 8 hours of sleep a night. Not only will you wake up feeling better, but you will also find that mentally you are more aware and sharp throughout the day.

There's nothing worse than walking into a client or account and looking like you haven't slept in days. You want to present yourself professionally—not like the walking dead. So do yourself a favor and make sleep a priority on your list of things to do.

Enjoy a massage

You work hard. Day in and day out you are sitting behind the wheel of your car. Depending on the size of your car, you could be cramped up all day long. This takes a toll on your body. You will find that your muscles are tighter (stiff neck or sore back) and ache. This is a sign that you need to get some work done on your muscles. More than likely you have numerous knots in your muscles (especially your back) that need to be worked out to get proper blood flow back into your muscles.

I recommend going to get a massage at least once a month. This will help you not only relax but it will help you relieve some stress. After the massage, make sure to drink plenty of water to help flush the toxins out of your body that were just broken up due to the massage.

Family first

This is something that is very important to those of you who have a family—whether it be just a husband/wife or a spouse with kids. You need to make sure your family comes first. No matter how much money you make out on the road, what you have at home is more important than anything else in the world—and you need to make sure they know that. We understand that you do what you do in order to support what's at home, but all the money in the world won't buy you a loving husband/wife and children.

When you come home on the weekends or whatever days you are off from work, you need to make sure that is your time with your family. Turn off the work smartphone, shut down your laptop, and enjoy that time with your family. Then when it's time to go back to work, get down to business. But your downtime is yours and you need that time to get away from work and go back to the things that keep you grounded.

If you find that work is interfering with your family, then you need to decide what means more to you—and hopefully, you know the correct answer to that. There needs to be some compromise. No employer should expect you to take time away from your family when not at work.

Traveling can be a fun time, don't get me wrong—you get to see a lot of interesting places during your travels. But make sure that work doesn't turn you away from your family. They need you just as much as you need your job. You simply need to find a happy medium between the two and be able to separate work time from family time.

Eating Smart While Traveling

Face it, some of us simply can't be stuck behind a desk all day long in a tiny cubicle staring at a computer monitor until our eyes cross. For those of you who are on the road majority of the year, I feel for you and I understand the stresses that come along with it. Some days you almost wish you were stationary typing away on your keyboard rather than staring through your windshield.

Besides the obvious stress of being away from home and your loved ones, you have to deal with traffic for 8+ hours a day, deal with changing weather conditions during those hours, find a place to sleep each night based on the area you are working, and the topic of this section— proper nutrition while working out of your car.

I've been in the fitness industry for quite some time now, and have been traveling regularly for over 6 years. Traveling isn't as bad as people make it out to be—you get to see new places, sightsee while traveling, and meet a lot of new people. The fork in the road comes when it's time to eat. Most people grab something quick at a fast-food restaurant—hence why a good portion of the US is overweight and obese. If you don't plan out each meal ahead of time you are setting yourself up for disaster.

Consider this section your roadmap to finding your way to a healthy body even when you feel like you took a couple of wrong turns on the way.

Let's start off with the essentials. You need to grocery shop and do it often. You should try and find a hotel that has a room with a refrigerator, freezer, oven, stove, and microwave. Personally, I enjoy staying at the Residence Inn (a Marriott property) if possible. They offer a full kitchen with a nice office/desk area to get work done.

Find the nearest grocery store once you get to the hotel. If they have a "bonus card" or something similar that offers you savings, sign up for one—the majority of them are free. More than likely during your travels you will run into another one of these grocery stores and the savings will definitely add up even after your first visit.

Fresh whole foods are always the way to go over supplements when you are able to fit them in. Protein shakes and bars are perfect for when you are in a pinch or want something quick between meals but you should still strive to fit in whole food meals if at all possible. If you want to fit in an extra 1-2 meals/snacks that consist of protein bars or shakes that would be fine. When grocery shopping try to pick up as much fresh food as you can. Remember, if you have a hotel room with a fridge, you can store these foods for the next day if you are there for more than one night. If you only stay there for one night you can buy just enough for that day/night and then grocery shop again the following day.

Or, you can use a portable mini fridge/warmer that can plug into your car. I personally have a Coleman car fridge which doubles as a warmer. I'm not telling you Coleman is the only way to go, but this is the one I purchased and I have no complaints. I am able to store my food in there that needs to be kept cold or I can set it to keep foods warm which I prepared that morning or the night before. This allows me to grab hot whole food meals while on the road and avoid fast food altogether. My model also has two cup holders as well where I can store some extra bottles of water.

If you are staying at a hotel which doesn't have an oven or stove, I highly recommend purchasing something like a George Foreman Grill so you can prepare your chicken/fish/beef products.   The same macronutrient choices mentioned earlier in the bulking tips section apply while traveling no matter if you are bulking or cutting.

In terms of hydration, I am a huge fan of water (seems like I'm a broken record on this throughout the book but water is so important for overall health and keeping your body functioning properly). No matter where I am I carry a gallon jug of water. I highly recommend that you do the same thing every day. Not only is water the best option in terms of what to drink in order to stay hydrated, but it is also free of calories, sugars, and carbohydrates.

Also, by using a gallon jug it allows you to monitor your water intake each day. You want to strive for at least a gallon a day. I will say this, when on the road and drinking a gallon of water, be prepared to make some extra bathroom breaks. Remember when I said stay away from fast-food chains when you are hungry, these locations are now an exception for when you need to hit the restroom. Get in and get out without ordering anything so you stick to your diet.

After a few weeks of being on the road and testing everything out, you will find yourself settling into your own routine and how to stay on track nutritionally while on the road. The key thing to remember is to plan ahead. If you don't plan ahead, then you are planning for failure.

Holiday Motivation

The below focuses on the holiday season and New Year's, but the same concepts can be followed for any holiday you celebrate.

When it's that time of the year, gyms will start filling up and all of those people with a fitness resolution will have their expectations soaring. Those who aren't already members of gyms will be out searching for the best of the best to join with all of their friends in hopes that they will all work out together. Little do they know that more than half of them will drop out within the first 90 days. It's no secret that the number one resolution for most people is to make fitness a priority and get in shape.

With high hopes and open wallets, they jump on the latest trends they see on TV or around town. January 1st hits and with all of their new workout clothes they got over the holidays they hit the gym—but with what purpose? Ah yes, something they weren't thinking about—they need a plan of attack! Without a plan of attack, it is like going into battle without any ammo, it will only get you so far.

For those who are already exercising and are members of a gym, the holidays are a busy time where for the majority of the people, exercise isn't on their holiday gift list. With all the hustle and bustle of the holiday, making cookies, decorating, being with family, extra time to take for yourself isn't as easy as some may wish. This section will hopefully give you some great ideas on how to stay on track during the holiday season, and for those who are just starting off, hopefully, this section will get you off on the right foot towards lifelong success and a healthier you.

How bad do you want it?

When it all comes down to it, the real question is—how badly do you want it? If you want it bad enough you will easily succeed. If you are motivated to start exercising and take control of your life, then you are one step ahead of everyone else. The hardest part is actually starting an exercise program. Once you start exercising and start seeing and feeling the benefits, you will easily be hooked for life.

Find something that motivates you and leave yourself reminders of why you need to keep on track. They can be something as simple as a word or a picture. Whatever you choose, put it somewhere that you will constantly be reminded of it. Some people who have issues with their diet put their motivation on their fridge, that way when they are hungry and go to get a snack, they see their motivation and rather than grabbing for that ice cream they grab for something healthy like veggies. This is also a great place to put your short and long-term goals that we spoke about earlier in this book. Half the battle is getting it implanted in your head that exercise has many benefits and that by exercising you are improving your health and taking control of your body.

If you want to lose weight, only you can get yourself there, no one else can do it for you. There's no magic pill and not something you can pay someone to do for you. It's not going to be easy, but you can achieve anything. If it were easy then everyone would be doing it. Exercise isn't a once and done thing, it is a lifestyle change. The term "lifestyle change" might scare some people, but by making small changes over time, switching from an unhealthy lifestyle to a healthy lifestyle won't seem so harsh. Again, it's all in your head. If you can overcome the urges to cheat on your diet or skip a workout, then the sky is the limit to your success and achieving your goals.

Create a plan before the New Year

Whether you are planning to start exercising for the New Year or are already on the path, it is wise to sit down and create a written plan for yourself. You want to write down some short and long-term goals. Make sure the goals are things that you can measure—this makes it much easier for you to track your progress.

If you hold off making a plan until after the New Year, you will be less likely to get started as people tend to keep pushing things off until eventually, they are forgotten about. If you truly want to live a longer, healthier life, then creating a plan early is your best bet to getting started and reaching your goals.

Eat throughout the day before a holiday party

No matter what the occasion, it is smart to eat throughout the day of a party (it doesn't even necessarily need to be a holiday, it could just be a celebration/party that friends or family are having). This will keep you full so when you go to the party you aren't starving and chow down on the food you shouldn't be eating. Also, by eating throughout the day, you will have a constant supply of nutrients to feed your muscles and help them grow and recover.

Eat healthy foods at the party

Your best bet when watching your weight during the holidays is to make sure you don't over-indulge at parties. It is very easy to step off the right path when you see all of that good (but unhealthy) food. Your food of choice while at a party should be focused on protein or vegetables if available. This can be lean meats, anything on a veggie tray, nuts, etc. Where most people get in trouble is with all the foods that are loaded with unhealthy carbs and fats.

Nuts are a great snack-type option to eat before or after a meal to create satiety. Anything from peanuts to almonds will do just fine. No nuts around other than some of your friends/relatives? Then veggies are your next best option. It's not uncommon to see carrots, celery, broccoli, and such as snacks laying around at gatherings. However, where you see veggies, you will also see dips. The smart move would be to stay away from the dips, as most of them are full of fats. If you must, put a little dip on your plate to eat with your veggies to give them some extra flavoring but don't overdo it.

The holidays bring families together but it also brings along pies and cakes. Load your plate with some proteins and healthy carbohydrates and dig in and enjoy yourself. The great thing about protein is that it fills you up fairly quickly and it also keeps you full longer. Another little trick is to drink water at a party. Water will help keep you feeling full and less likely to grab a whole plate of cookies and disappear into another room of the house only to devour the entire plate.

<u>Schedule workouts</u>

During the holidays in order to make sure you get a workout in, you need to schedule some time in your day. Pick the days you want to work out and write in exactly what time you want to exercise and make sure those plans don't change. Without scheduling your workouts, it is easy (especially during the holidays) to find yourself doing something else rather than exercising.

With so much to do, people tend to use the excuse that they don't have time to fit in workouts during the holidays. Having no time is one of the oldest excuses in the book. Waking up a little earlier in the morning to get in a workout really isn't that hard to do once you get a routine down.

A lot of people also work out on lunch breaks in order to get their workout in. Some people just do cardio on lunch breaks while others try and get in a quick weight workout. If people are lucky enough to get an hour lunch break, it gives most people enough time to do a weight workout along with some cardio. The main point to take from this is simple—it doesn't matter how you do it or when you do it, just make sure you schedule a time to exercise.

<u>Work out in the mornings</u>

The best time of the day to get a workout in would definitely be in the morning. By doing a workout in the morning, you are opening the rest of the day to whatever you need to get done. Also, by working out in the morning, you're less likely to miss your workout because you got caught up in the middle of something else and had to change your plans. By starting the day off on the right foot with a workout, your metabolism is already jump-started and you will be burning more calories throughout the day. It's a win-win.

Exercise at home

We all know holidays are super busy and that most gyms aren't open on certain holidays. So what do you do when this happens? You improvise and work out at home! Sure you aren't going to have access to heavy dumbbells, a wide variety of machines, and rows and rows of cardio machines—but you don't have to have all that fancy stuff! Heck no, you can get a decent workout right in your own home. Now I'm not saying this is a type of workout that you should do all the time (not unless you cannot afford a gym membership or some home equipment). But when you are rushed for time and you need to get a workout in, you can literally hit every body part one way or another right in the comfort of your own home.

You can easily find things around your house to use to get in a workout. You could do things such as pushups, crunches, sit-ups, close-grip pushups, biceps curls (with weighted objects around the house), shoulder presses (with weighted objects around the house), bodyweight squats, and bent over rows (with weighted objects around the house) in order to get in a workout. For cardio, you can simply go for a walk or jog and if you have access to a bike you could even go for a nice bike ride.

For those of you who already have a gym membership, it still wouldn't be a bad idea to get yourself some inexpensive pieces of equipment for at home in case you need to fit in a quick workout and driving to the gym and back would not make sense. This can be anything from resistance bands to adjustable compact dumbbells. You don't need a ton of equipment or a lot of space to get in a great workout at home.

Some people financially cannot afford to work out in a gym—not a problem. Equipment can be purchased for use at home. Another great thing about having equipment that you can use at home would be that you have no excuse that you didn't have time to go to the gym since the gym is already in your home. You don't have to spend time on the road driving to and from the gym and you don't have to wait till someone is done using a machine. By having a gym at your house you can find a time during the day that is convenient for you and get a quick workout in.

Exercise with the family

A great source of motivation is right where you need it the most—at home with your family. If you are the only person (or one of the few people) in your family that works out, a great way to get others started slowly would be to include them in your exercise program. During the holidays after most people stuff their faces and then lay around on the couch wishing they didn't eat so much. A great way to burn off those extra calories you just ate is to take a walk—and take your family with you.

A nice walk in the park or around the block will suffice. You don't want to go for a marathon of a walk which will more than likely deter your family from exercising again in the future. The plan here isn't to scare them away, but to show them how much fun it can be to exercise. If they enjoy the walk together, ask them to go through a weight workout with you—explain to them the benefits of exercise. Who knows, you might be just the person to get your family kick-started into exercising and you could be the motivation that helps them reach their goals and live a healthier life.

Keep an exercise journal

The best way to track your progress is to write each of your workouts down in an exercise journal. Chart every exercise, set, rep, type and duration of cardio, and the date. Your exercise journal can be anything from a notepad to a piece of computer paper, to a chart you made on the computer. The key here is to be consistent with writing down your workouts and making sure you aren't taking steps backward.

By keeping a journal, you have something can go back in time and see exactly how you have been progressing over the past couple of weeks, months, and even years. Another great advantage of keeping an exercise journal is if and when you get to a sticking point you can look back in your journal and see what you did the last time to get you out of that plateau.

The people who don't keep a journal never know exactly how they are progressing because they have no way of measuring what they accomplished in the past. By writing everything down you can go back to the week before and make sure you aren't using a weight that is less than what was used previously or that you didn't cut yourself short on a piece of cardio equipment. The time spent writing everything in the journal during your workouts (which takes no time at all since most people write things in the journal while resting between sets) is well worth the knowledge and progression you will see down the road.

Walk extra when shopping

Need to get some cardio in but you have to go shopping and don't have thirty minutes to an hour to run to the gym to get it in? Not a problem! The answer is quite simple—do your cardio while shopping. No that doesn't mean wear your cut off t-shirt or sports bra while shopping, nor does it mean for you to run up and down the aisles like a maniac flinging sweat on everyone. All you have to do is walk. That means don't drive around the mall looking for the closest parking space. Instead, you should park far away from the doors and walk—as in the back of the parking lot.

Then while in the mall or anywhere you need to go shopping, take the stairs if you have to change floors rather than using the elevator (assuming where you are shopping has multiple levels). You can even walk the mall or shopping area at a fast pace to elevate your heart rate more.

Shovel snow rather than using a snowblower

Snowed in and can't run to the gym for a workout? Don't start up that snowblower, instead grab a shovel (assuming you are healthy enough to do so). Shoveling involves many muscle groups and depending on how much you have to shovel, you can actually get in a pretty good workout. Obviously, if you have heart conditions or are getting up in age, I recommend for your health and safety that you use the snow blower or at least talk to your doctor about if shoveling could cause any adverse effects to your health. But for those looking to get a workout in, shoveling is your best bet.

If you don't have a lot of snow to shovel (maybe your driveway is small) and you are in a helpful mood, shovel your neighbor's driveway and sidewalk as well or help someone shovel their car out so they can get to work or where they need to go. Shoveling snow not only gets your strength training workout in, but you also burned a decent amount of calories as well. This is a clear win-win situation for you on a snow day.

Avoid extra calories on alcohol

Alcohol not only adds extra calories to your diet, but it also lowers testosterone which is needed to help build lean muscle mass. Those couple drinks that you have a party can easily add up to well over 1,000 calories by the time the night is over (assuming you are of drinking age). Guess what happens to those added calories? They get stored as FAT! Something you don't want to happen, especially during the holidays when you're trying to look your best. The worst part is, those people mixing drinks, not only are you getting your extra calories which you don't need from the alcohol, but also from the soda you are using to mix your drink with. And beer, yes, we are all aware that people love to drink beer.

It is in your best interest to lower beer/alcohol consumption especially if you want to see better progress with your fitness goals. Your best bet is to either drink water or tea (your best option would definitely be water) during holiday parties or maybe have one drink and sip on it throughout the night.

Drink plenty of water

Water not only keeps you hydrated, but it is also a zero-calorie beverage. A much better choice when compared to what most people are consuming during the holidays. With calorie-filled adult beverages and alcohol flowing during these times, it is hard to say no to the temptation. However, if you are truly set on reaching your fitness goals, you must stick with the plan and reach for the water. If you decide to have some drinks, it is best to spread them out over a couple days of parties you will be attending and to "nurse" the drink so you aren't tempted to quickly drink it and get another one.

By drinking plenty of water you will also feel fuller throughout the day so you will be less likely to binge on foods that you shouldn't be eating between meals. This not only cuts down on your calorie intake, but it also makes sure you are properly hydrated to keep your metabolism fired up.

Supplements: What you NEED Versus What you WANT

Money-Saving Supplement Choices

Let's face it, things these days aren't cheap. The prices of homes are on the rise, food is getting more expensive, and overall the cost of living is always rising. Well, the same thing goes with supplements. The cost of raw materials is rising and with everyone and their brother trying to get into the industry which is driving up the demand for the raws, it's no wonder these suppliers have hiked the price up.

With so many choices out there on the market, it is tough to pick what would benefit you the most. You have salesmen trying to persuade you to purchase something that will give them a nice commission, your friends are telling you to try something they used, you see all the ads in magazines and online—what exactly do you need? There are just too many choices with a lot of different price ranges. Well, I'm here to shed some light on the subject and help you reach your goals without breaking your bank account.

There are the basics that everyone should be using, and then there are accessory supplements. The basics are the things that you

SHOULD have in order to stay healthy and also to make any type of lean mass gains.

Accessory supplements are things that you can add to your supplement arsenal if you have some extra money. These products don't necessarily give you any gains; most of them are a temporary feeling such as vasodilatation products, which give you a nice pump while in the gym. None of these products will be mentioned in this book.

<u>Here is a list of the basics that you should pick up (in no particular order):</u>

- Protein Powder
- Multivitamin
- Fish Oil
- Creatine

Now I'm sure you are wondering why I chose these products. Below is my reasoning. But first, be sure to talk to your doctor before adding any supplements to your regimen to ensure they will not react with any other medications or health issues you have.

Protein Powder

Protein powder is a cheap and fairly inexpensive way to increase your daily intake of protein. There are men out there who simply can't eat enough whole food protein sources to reach their 160+ grams of protein each day. Majority of the protein powders on the market have a great nutrition profile and will fill in any gap you are lacking during the day. They can be used as a snack or even as meal replacements if you can't fit in a whole food meal. However, the main use of protein powders should be for post-workout nutrition. You want to feed your muscles around 20-40 grams of protein after your workout to give them the nutrients they need to repair and grow. There are many different types of protein powder out there so find one that meets your needs and one that you enjoy the taste.

Your best choice for a protein powder is whey. It can either be a concentrate or an isolate. Concentrate will be less expensive. The isolates tend to be more expensive because they are absorbed better and faster than concentrates. Isolates are also lower in carbohydrates compared to whey concentrate powders. If the price is an issue, a concentrate is your best choice. Whey concentrate is generally recommended for most beginners due to its flexibility of use and lower price point. Some people do, however, mention they have digestive issues while using concentrates. Everyone is different, so see how it works for you. You can always try out an isolate at a later time.

There are also slow-digesting proteins called casein, which is great to use before bed. Casein digests between 5-7 hours which makes it ideal for at night before bed since you won't get eating for roughly 8 hours. By throwing in some casein protein at night your body will stay anabolic and build and repair muscle rather than halting the recovery process.

Multivitamin

A multivitamin is probably the most important aspect to anyone no matter if they are exercising or not. In order for your body to work properly, it needs the proper vitamins and minerals to do so. If you become deficient in any area, your health and performance will decline. Each vitamin and mineral assists with thousands of biochemical reactions in the body and help keep hormone levels steady. So what does all of this mean? It means if you don't use a multivitamin or you use a cheap one, you won't get the results you are looking for.

Fish Oil

Fish oil is a great source of Omega-3 fatty acids as well as EFA's (essential fatty acids). A good fish oil should include EPA and DHA. These are the "good fats" that we all need. They help lower cholesterol and also improve cardiovascular health—not to mention all of the cancer and illness prevention you can get from the fish oil. It also helps improve joint flexibility as well as supporting brain, nerve, and visual functioning. Fish oil can be found in liquid form (which most people don't like the taste of) and also in pill form which is the preferred method by most people.

Creatine

For those of you who are interested in the human body should already know that creatine is naturally found in all of our bodies. Its use is to give us energy to do quick explosive movements. It gives us creatine phosphate (CP), which then breaks apart and rebuilds to form ATP, which produces more energy as fuel for our muscles. Creatine is what helps us keep the intensity up in our workout without hitting the wall early on. It also helps us recover faster not only during our workout but after our workout (which is when we grow).

Creatine is found in our bodies as I stated above, and it is also found in some of the foods that we eat—including red meat as well as in fish. However, in order to get the dosage that you need, you would have to eat a lot of red meat and fish, which doesn't make sense and would be mighty expensive. Creatine can be found in tablet or pill form and also in a powder. There are plain creatine monohydrate products as well as micronized creatine, CEE, and creatine HCl products. All of which basically do the same thing.

The least expensive creatine out on the market today is creatine monohydrate. Some people are non-responders to creatine, so it might not work for everyone. However, if you get small gains off of the monohydrate, you can try out the different types of creatine to see what works best for your body. There is no one supplement that works for everyone—all of our bodies are unique and react differently to supplements.

Creatine does not need to be loaded and it is a personal preference if you want to cycle it or not. You can safely take creatine both before and after your workouts. For those who cycle creatine, you will find that you will lose a little weight when you cycle off—no it's not muscle mass you lost! Creatine by nature causes water to flood your cells and muscles. When you stop using creatine for a period of time, some of the water that flooded your muscles and cells will be diminished.

With all the products that are out there, I hope this opened your eyes to exactly what you NEED to have rather than what you WANT to have.

Not only is this going to save you money, but also this will help you achieve the muscle mass you always wanted. If you have some extra money left over and you want to experiment with other products such as pre and intra-workout supplementation, by all means, go ahead and try them. Just be aware that the effects that you will get from most products outside of what is mentioned above will diminish and fade away when they are stopped. Remember, you need a good basic foundation before you can build a house.

The Importance of Hydration

Water

Many people overlook the benefits of hydration. There are those who do not like the taste of water, therefore they drink soda, tea, coffee, etc. No matter what the excuse, they are missing out on the most important factor in overall health. There are many different types of water that can be purchased and like anything else, there are sources that are better than others. This section will shed some light on the importance of water and what sources are best.

What is so important about water?

The human body cannot make or store water so it is necessary to drink water throughout the day to replace what you eliminated. Water makes up about 60 percent of our total body weight and is involved in almost every bodily process.

How much water do we need to drink?

As a rule of thumb, everyone should strive to drink around a gallon of water each day. You can also figure out how much water you need to drink in a round-about way by taking your body weight in pounds and multiplying it by 0.55 to figure out how many ounces you need. So a

200-pound individual would need 110 ounces of water a day (200 x 0.55 = 110). Obviously, if you are an athlete or avid exerciser, you will need more water so you can replace what you lost during a workout or practice.

For those who exercise or play sports, drink plenty of fluids before, during, and after the activity to avoid overheating and to stay hydrated. You want to replace whatever fluids you lost due to exercise as soon as possible following each session.

You want to be drinking even when you aren't thirsty. By the time you are thirsty, you have already become slightly dehydrated. On average, when you have lost about 2% of your body weight from water is when you will start to feel thirsty. By this time, it is too late and performance (especially in sports) will decline. Continue to drink even after you are satisfied. If you stop when you are satisfied, you will actually only get about half the amount you really needed.

<u>Will any water do the trick?</u>

When exercising under 60 minutes, cool water is the best fluid to keep you hydrated. For events lasting longer than 60 minutes, a sports drink that contains 6-10% carbohydrates will be ideal.

It is important that you don't drink just any kind of water. You want to be careful where you are getting your source from. You want to make sure the water you drink is pure so that you aren't flooding your body with toxic chemicals. Tap water for one normally contains chlorine, radon, arsenic, as well as other toxic chemicals that are not healthy.

It is best to purchase filtered water from a grocery store or if you prefer to save money by using tap water, at a minimum you need to purchase a good high-quality filtration system. This filtration system can be as complex or as simple as you wish. You can install an in-home filtration system that is hooked up to the waterline in your home. You can also attach a filtration system to the faucet of your sink. This device allows you to switch between filtered and unfiltered so when you are washing dishes and didn't want to blow through the filter, you can turn the knob on the filtration device to allow it to pass through without running through the filtration device.

Another option would be a water pitcher that has a filtration device in it. It's actually quite simple but you'll find yourself filling it up quite often if you go this route. What you do is put water into filtration device on the pitcher and it slowly works its way through the proprietary filtration system and what is left at the bottom of the container is the filtered water. Very simple.

No matter which way you decide to go, you will need to change your filters by following the recommended guidelines provided by the manufacturer of the device or filtration system. This will ensure your water is as pure as possible before drinking.

Does water from food count in daily requirements?

Good news for those who eat a lot of raw plant foods! If you are eating a large number of plant foods, your daily water requirement will already have a decent amount fulfilled by those foods. Plant foods are primarily 80% water. But the answer is still no. You shouldn't count water from food in your daily requirement. I would recommend still drinking close to a gallon of water each day in addition to your plant-based foods to ensure proper hydration throughout the day.

Water cleanses the body!

In the world of the fitness industry, high protein diets are what make up a large percentage of the population. With that being said, the body needs to cleanse itself from the urea and ketones, which is brought on by high protein consumption. It is necessary to get rid of all these toxins in the body to help the kidneys function optimally.

Will water help me lose weight?

You bet it will! I know what you are thinking, that if you drink a lot of water you will get bloated and retain water, which will make you weigh more. However, this isn't the case. If you aren't drinking enough water, your body will hold on to whatever water is already in your body and will not excrete any. This means the water in your body will be used for normal bodily functions and will cause you to appear bloated. The only way to get rid of that bloated look is to actually drink more water. By doing so, your body will function much better and your metabolism will start to increase and will help you burn calories more efficiently.

If you want to burn even more calories while drinking water, then you want to make sure the water is ice cold. Your body needs to warm up the water in order for it to be used properly. Warming up the water uses energy, which uses calories. This, in turn, will help you burn extra calories throughout the day. Now let's be clear, drinking ice cold water isn't going to be the new weight loss miracle. However, it will help you burn some extra calories throughout the day if utilized.

Feeling bloated?

If you are feeling and looking bloated, check your sodium intake. If you look in the mirror and find yourself holding onto water, you need to either lower your sodium intake or increase your water intake. What would I recommend? Doing both.

What are some tips for staying hydrated?

- Weigh yourself before and after your workouts and drink 2-3 cups of water for every pound of weight you lost during your workout. You want to have your body weight back to normal before your next workout.

- Drink small amounts of water frequently rather than large amounts less often.

- Pay attention to the amount and color of your urine. You should excrete urine that is nearly colorless. Small amounts of dark-colored urine can indicate dehydration.

- Drink cold beverages to cool your core body temperature and reduce sweating.

- Carry a water bottle with you at all times to ensure you can drink throughout the day.

- Start and end your day with water. Your body loses water while you sleep so by drinking some when you first wake and when you go to bed you will ensure proper hydration.

- When struck by the flu or a cold, you will become dehydrated and should always keep water by your side at all time.

Can I die from drinking too much water?

Unfortunately, yes. I am sure most of you have heard about the incident that happened in California where a lady entered a contest at a radio station to win a Nintendo Wii (that game system seems so old now, guess that's a sign I'm getting old too). The radio station held a contest where contestants drank as much water as they could without going to the bathroom and the last person still in the contest would win the new game system. She placed second in the contest but became very ill. The lady then died in her home of water intoxication.

This is rare but it can happen. What happens is that when too much water enters the cells, the tissues swell. This causes an electrolyte and salt imbalance which can cause irregular heartbeat and allow fluid to enter the lungs. The pressure due to swelling will also put pressure on the brain and nerves, which can also cause problems. Swelling in the brain can cause coma, seizures, and even death.

What it really comes down to is not so much how much you drink, but the time frame in which you drank all the water. The body can take in up to fifteen liters of water a day—which most people will never reach. However, in a small time frame that can be dangerous. It is said that consuming 0.79 gallons of water at one sitting can be fatal for someone who adheres to a normal diet (not low in sodium and not exercising prior to drinking).

Seasonality Health and Fitness Secrets

- **Summer Weight Loss**
- **Cold Weather Workouts**

Summer Weight Loss

Find yourself dreading the thought of putting on your swimsuit? The time is now to get yourself ready for the beach and the nice warm summer weather. Show off all the hard work you put in at the gym by shedding off those extra pounds you added over the winter months while bulking. Below you will find some helpful tips to help you get ready for the summer.

1) Ditch the junk!

Say goodbye to McDonalds and Wendy's and say hello to homemade cooking. This should be a no-brainer but people still think that if they go to the gym they can eat whatever they want. WRONG! If you seriously want to shape up for the summer, you need to kiss fast food joints goodbye. Not only are these places loaded with calories but also the fat content is through the roof.

If you haven't watched the movie *Supersize Me*, you need to go rent it today and watch it. If you don't get sick watching that movie and seeing for yourself that McDonalds' French fries can last well over three months without sprouting any mold, then you honestly don't have all systems firing upstairs.

To be totally honest, eating out at a restaurant isn't much different than eating at a fast-food chain. Normal portion sizes when eating out are way more than what you need per meal. So unless you plan on creating two portions from anything you get when eating out at a restaurant, you are going to end up well over your calories for the day.

I also recommend requesting to have things prepared a certain way. Rather than having vegetables prepared in butter, ask them to make it steamed without butter. Looking to enjoy a nice juicy steak or chicken breast? Most places put butter on them when preparing to add more flavor. Ask for everything to be made without butter and steamed/grilled to keep the calories down.

Also, watch what they put in your salad. Many places load up on the cheese and croutons as well as dressings that are high in fat. I'd recommend skipping the croutons altogether. In terms of the cheese, if you really want it I'd ask for it on the side as well as your dressing so you can add just a tiny amount of each to your salad.

2) Cook at home

When eating out you never really know how your food is prepared unless you ask them to prepare your food a certain way. Therefore, your best bet is to prepare and cook your own food. When you eat out many of the foods you are ingesting are cooked in butter or other fattening ingredients, which is exactly the stuff you want to stay away from. Do we even need to get into all the fried foods that are out there? You want to talk about a heart attack waiting to happen… fried foods throw up the red light. STAY AWAY! Your best bet for cooking at home can be anything from grilling your foods, steaming your foods, and even baking your foods.

Portion sizes are another issue with eating out. When you eat out and see the food on your plate, your natural instinct is to finish everything on your plate. Did you stop to think about how many calories you just took in eating that whole plate? Probably not. This is a quick and easy fix by simply preparing all of your food at home. Not only will you know exactly how your food is prepared, but you can make sure everything is portioned out correctly.

The American Cancer Society created a great visual to ensure proper portion control by naming objects that correspond to correct portion sizes:

- 1 oz. meat: the size of a matchbox
- 3 oz. meat: the size of a deck of cards or bar of soap
- 8 oz. meat: the size of a thin paperback book
- 3 oz. fish: the size of a checkbook
- 1 oz. cheese: the size of 4 dice
- Medium potato: the size of a computer mouse
- 2 Tbsp. peanut butter: the size of a ping pong ball
- 1 cup pasta: the size of a tennis ball
- Average bagel: the size of a hockey puck
- Medium apple or orange: the size of a tennis ball
- 1 cup chopped raw vegetables or fruit: baseball size
- 1/4 cup dried fruit (raisins, apricots, mango): a small handful
- Lunch-box size container of unsweetened applesauce
- Cup of lettuce: four leaves

Also, when you are eating at home, make sure you aren't eating from a bag. The worst thing you can do is continually reach into a bag and keep eating and not know how much you consumed. After no time at all, you can throw down a couple hundred calories and not even know it. Always take products out of the bag and portion it so you can track how much of something you ate.

3) Where's the beef?

When looking to lose weight the best thing you can do (especially when weight training) is to increase your protein intake while cutting out some of your carbs. This protein source can be anything from natural foods to protein shakes and bars.

4) Watch your carbs and watch your spare tire disappear

This is pretty much common sense… if you eat a bunch of carbs you can sit back and watch your stomach grow. There are good carbs and then there are bad carbs. Feel free to eat fruits and vegetables and not feel bad about it. The red flag should appear when you start drooling over cakes, white flour products, pasta, and things of that nature. Those products can pack on the calories in a hurry.

You want to concentrate on carbs that are low glycemic rather than high glycemic. Low glycemic carbohydrates will raise and lower your blood sugar slowly while the high glycemic carbohydrates will make your blood sugar spike quickly and then crash.

Low glycemic diets will:

- reduce hunger and keep you fuller for longer
- help people lose and control weight
- increase the body's sensitivity to insulin
- improve diabetes control
- prolong physical endurance
- help re-fuel carbohydrate stores after exercise
- reduce the risk of heart disease
- reduce blood cholesterol levels

<u>Here is a list of some great choices from the low GI list:</u>

- All-bran
- Apple juice
- Apples
- Apricots (dried)
- Artichoke
- Asparagus
- Baked beans, tinned
- Bananas
- Barley, cracked
- Black-eyed beans
- Broccoli
- Carrot juice
- Carrots, cooked
- Cauliflower
- Celery
- Cherries
- Chickpeas

- Chickpeas, tinned
- Cucumber
- Eggplant
- Grapefruit
- Grapefruit juice
- Grapes
- Green beans
- Kidney beans, boiled
- Kidney beans, tinned
- Kiwi fruit
- Lentil soup, tinned
- Lentils green, boiled
- Lentils green, tinned
- Lettuce, all varieties
- Low-fat yogurt, artificially sweetened
- Milk, skimmed
- Milk, chocolate
- Milk, fat-free
- Milk, semi-skimmed
- Milk, whole
- Multi-grain bread
- Orange juice
- Oranges
- Peaches
- Peanuts
- Pearl barley
- Pears
- Peas, dried
- Peppers, all varieties
- Pineapple juice
- Plums
- Rye

- Snow peas
- Soya beans, boiled
- Soya milk
- Spaghetti, protein-enriched
- Spaghetti, whole wheat
- Spinach
- Sweet potato
- Tomato soup, tinned
- Tomatoes
- Wheat kernels
- Whole grain
- Yam
- Yogurt low-fat (sweetened)
- Young summer squash
- Zucchini

5) Drink up, sailor!

Water that is. Water should become your new best friend if you haven't already become acquainted. Sodas and similar drinks are loaded with sugars and empty calories that should be avoided at all costs. Those extra calories add up over the course of a couple months and make you gain unwanted weight.

It is extremely important to replenish water after a workout. Not only can you suffer from dehydration (especially in hot weather), but becoming deficient of water can cause normal bodily functions to either not work efficiently or can make them shut down—both cases not being ideal.

A simple way to figure out how many ounces of water you need a day is to simply take your body weight in pounds and multiply it by 0.55.

Example: Say you weigh 170 pounds
          (170 x 0.55) = 93.5 ounces of water

Don't like doing math? Then strive for around a gallon of water each day.

6) Weight training

I think it is pretty much understood these days that in order to lose weight you need to do some sort of weight training. Weight training benefits everyone, ranging from kids to the elderly.

<u>What can weight training do for you?</u>

- Increases strength
- Increases endurance
- Increases metabolism
- Relieves stress
- Increases and restores bone density
- Reduces the risk of osteoporosis
- Increases lean muscle mass
- Prevents injuries
- Improves balance
- Decreases the risk of disease

- Enhances sport performance
- Improves body image
- Lowers blood pressure
- Lowers resting heart rate
- Elevates mood
- Burns fat

So what's not to love about weight training? With all the benefits mentioned above and many more out there, you would be foolish to leave this out of your summer prep let alone your daily life. With as little as two days a week of weight training, you can significantly change your physique and your life by adding this to your regimen. Of course, if you can get in 3-4 days of weight training a week that would be even better.

Weight training can either be done in full-body workouts or they can be split up into certain muscles groups each day. Either way you choose to train will be effective in helping you reach your summer weight loss goals.

Ladies… remember, no matter how much weight you lift you will never get as big as the guys in the gym. Don't let that be a factor that steers you away from weight training. Men naturally have more testosterone which allows them to build muscle much quicker than females. So go to the gym and don't be afraid to pick up some heavy weights, they don't bite. Who knows, you might even be able to show up some of the guys in the gym!

7) Cardio sucks!

Let's face it, cardio sucks. There isn't any way around it, but it has to be done. The key is to find something that you enjoy doing and go with it. This can be anything from playing sports to something as simple as walking around the neighborhood. Whatever the case may be, find that something that you enjoy doing that raises your heart rate into the target zone (strive for between 60-70% of your heart rate max).

In order to find your target heart rate, use the formulas below:

(220 – your age – your resting HR) x 0.60 + your resting HR = your HR at 60% your max

(220 – your age – your resting HR) x 0.70 + your resting HR = your HR at 70% your max

Example: Say you are 32 years old and your resting heart rate is 63.

(220 – 32 – 63) x 0.60 + 63 = 138 at 60%
(220 – 32 – 63) x 0.70 + 63 = 151 at 70%

Therefore, you want to have your heart rate between 138 and 151 when you are doing your cardio. Math, not your thing? Look for a heart rate monitor that allows you to input all of your personal data which then, in turn, will be able to calculate without you needing to do anything, your target heart rate. Very simple but will cost you a little more than a basic heart rate monitor that does nothing more than read your heart rate.

8) Make a list and check it twice

No, it's not Christmas and I'm not Santa Claus (bummer, I know)… But now is the time to write down some goals that you want to accomplish. You should have both short-term and long-term goals down on paper. The short-term goals can either be weekly weight loss goals or monthly weight loss goals that take you into the summer. The long-term goals you set should take you a couple of months down the road if not over a year.

When setting weight loss goals, take into consideration that you can lose 1-2 pounds a week. If you are losing more than that in a week's time you risk losing muscle mass which you don't want to do. So when looking at a month for a timeframe, you can lose 4-8 pounds a month and do it in a healthy manner.

9) Evaluate your goals

After a period of time, sit down with the list of goals you made and evaluate where you are at that given moment. If you find one of your goals is going to be a long shot, then change it to something more realistic. The point of making goals isn't to make them so hard that they are unobtainable, but to make them so you have a game plan for success. A timeline so to speak for your journey. Of course, you don't want to make them too easy, yet you don't want to make it something that you can never accomplish in a given amount of time. So go over your game plan often and make sure you are on track for success. If you aren't, sit down and re-evaluate. As long as you are on track, you will be ready for summer in no time.

10)   Have fun!

To me, this is the most important aspect of getting ready for the summer and dropping those last couple pounds that you might have put on during the winter months. You need to find something that you enjoy doing. If cardio on a treadmill isn't your thing, but you enjoy playing basketball—then, by all means, play basketball for your cardio. The same goes for weight training, if you don't like something then switch it up to a form of weight training that you enjoy.

Exercising and losing weight doesn't just to improve your health, it also helps you live a less stressful life—giving you the total mind, body, spirit experience.

Cold Weather Workouts

Depending on what part of the world you live in, you might see some of that white stuff falling from the sky that we all like to call, SNOW. With that being said, along with snow comes the possibility of ice. Both individually are dangerous when traveling, and together can be a deadly combination to those venturing out and about. Those diehard gym rats who will travel no matter what the weather is like will more than likely be one of the few at the gym during snowy/icy days.

So what do you do on those snowy/icy days? Sit in front of the television and eat a bag of potato chips? I sure hope not. Even though the weather outside isn't the greatest, that doesn't mean that you can't get a good workout in at home.

This section will give you some tips and pointers on how you can make your snowed-in day work for you and allow you to still get in a great workout.

Grab your shovel!

I know… We all hate going outside to shovel. What a "chore". The thought of going out to shovel snow ranks up there with watching paint dry. However, it doesn't have to be that way if you truly want a good full-body workout. Shoveling snow can burn on average anywhere from 300-500 calories per hour (that doesn't mean shoveling for 10 minutes and then standing there admiring your work for the other 50).

If you are no longer a spring chicken or you have health issues, make sure to check with your doctor first to make sure you are able to safely shovel snow. If not, then pay someone to shovel your driveway/walkway or invest in a snowblower.

For those of you who can shovel with no issues, feel free to help out your neighbors, especially around the holidays. Do the sidewalks all the way down your street, or help your next-door neighbor shovel out their driveway or car. Those extra burned calories add up. Say it takes you 1 hour to do your driveway, and then you help your neighbor do his/her driveway for an hour. That means you burned anywhere from 600-1000 calories just from shoveling. Doesn't sound so bad after all, right?

Home workouts

For those of you who have a home gym, you have no excuse to skip a workout (especially when it snows). You don't have to have a huge home gym to get in a good workout.

Those looking for a home gym outside of the resistance band route, here are the necessities that I would recommend (assuming you are invested in exercising for the duration of your life):

- power rack or smith machine
- barbell with weight set (300-pound set would be ideal)
- dumbbells (if worried about space invest in the adjustable weight version)
- adjustable bench

As you can see, you don't need a lot of things, just the basics will be enough to hit every body part. Some people can even get away with just having dumbbells and a bench. Either way, there is no excuse not to get in a good workout even on the coldest, wintry days of the year.

For those who have a stricter budget and cannot afford some or all of the equipment above, do not fear! Resistance bands are a very inexpensive way to fit in a workout using something other than household objects that are just heavy enough to give you some resistance. You can hit every muscle group with many different angles and exercises with these bands. They are also small enough to travel with you if you go on vacation or out of town.

Walk it off

Even though the weather outside is frightful (ok, let's not break out into the song "Let It Snow"), you can still take a nice walk outside assuming there isn't too much snow or ice. Bundle up with layers and make sure you are fully covered so you don't catch frostbite. Make sure you wear shoes with good tread so you have good traction. If it is a little icy outside, you can still go for a walk; you just need to be extra careful.

If you have snowshoes, you have it made. Take your walk off-road. If you have access to wooded areas around where you live, you can take a nice walk through the woods and check out the beautiful winter scenery. If you don't have access to the woods, take a nice walk through your entire neighborhoods backyards and wave to all your neighbors as they watch you through their windows (ok, this is a joke... please do not do this). But seriously, if you have snowshoes, your walk is endless and you can pretty much go wherever you wish. So get out and explore!

Cold weather actually burns more calories!

The nice thing about being outside when the weather is cold is that you burn more calories. Who would have thought that you could literally stand still in the winter outside and burn calories? Want to know why? Sure you do! Your body is programmed to maintain a temperature of 98.6 degrees Fahrenheit or 37.0 degrees Celsius. With that being said, your core temperature drops when you are outside. Therefore, your body needs to exert energy to bring the temperature back up (this can be in the form of shivering) which burns calories. I'm not saying that by standing outside you will lose 10 pounds, but you WILL burn a small number of calories simply by being out in the cold.

Do I recommend this for weight loss? No. How boring is that! But it is a fun fact to make you think about how the body burns calories and exerts energy, which increases the body's core temperature. There's your fun fact of the day!

Skiing/Snowboarding

Enjoy the slopes? Great! Skiing and snowboarding is a great way to get out in the winter and burn calories. Not to mention a fun way to take your mind off how cold it is and have a little fun in the process.

The great thing about skiing and snowboarding is that you go through a whole-body workout and don't even realize it. You are constantly using your legs and arms to make turns and go faster while your core is working nonstop to keep you from falling over and losing your balance. Some people even experience soreness the day after hitting the slopes, which isn't uncommon. A full day on the slopes is a great workout and can be done with the whole family.

Build a snowman or a snow fort

Looking for another idea for the whole family? Why not build a snowman or a snow fort? Heck, you could even have a snowball fight (watch the face when throwing snowballs, we don't want any injuries).

Walking around and carrying snowballs/snow-blocks burns calories and also gives you a strength workout. Large snowballs or snow-blocks get heavy and after carrying them around for some time and will definitely give you a good workout. Constantly placing the blocks on top of each other and moving them around is enough to stimulate and exhaust the muscle. The same goes for lifting large balls of snow and placing them on each other to form your snowman.

This is a good activity to give your whole family a workout and have some fun and family time in the process. Then when you are all done you can go inside and throw down some hot chocolate (which is full of antioxidants).

BONUS! Quick Nutrition Guide

- **Nutrition Guide**
- **Healthy Food List Reference**

Nutrition Guide

(Quick facts and overview of proper nutrition)

- Eat in moderation- take in 3-6 meals depending on how many "snack" meals you have during the day (breakfast-snack-lunch-snack-dinner-snack)

- Protein is the key ingredient to dieting because it acts as a stabilizer for sugars. Protein slows down the process that glucose, sugar, travels into the bloodstream. It rebuilds muscle tissue, burns fat for energy, provides calcium, vitamin A, B2, B12, strengthens the immune system, appetite suppressant, and improves the growth of hair, nails, and skin. Around 35% of your calories should come from protein. Recommended sources: egg whites, white chicken meat, turkey, any fish, low-fat or fat-free cheese, low-fat or fat-free cottage cheese, protein bars, and protein shakes to name a few. As a guide for meats, use the palm of your hand or a deck of cards to determine the serving size. Whenever eating a carbohydrate, always eat a protein with it.

- Carbohydrates are sugars that provide energy, better concentration, and a good source of fiber. Around 45% of your calories should come from carbohydrates. Fibrous Carbohydrates are fruits and vegetables which are a natural source that is full of nutritional value and should always be included in your daily diet.

- Fats provide essential fatty acids, energy, an appetite suppressant; good fats help our bodies release and break down the bad fats. If your daily fat intake is cut back too much, your body will preserve fat for survival rather than release it for energy.

- Protein: 1 gram = 4 calories

- Carbohydrates: 1 gram = 4 calories

- Fat: 1 gram = 9 calories

- Ratio: 45% Carbs – 35% Protein - 20% Fat

- 3,500 calories make up 1 pound of fat

- If you cut out 500 calories from your diet each day, you could potentially save/lose 1 pound a week. If you cut out 1,000 calories from your diet each day, you could potentially save/lose 2 pounds a week. It is not a good idea to be losing more than 2 pounds each week.

- Remember, resistance training boosts your metabolism while cardiovascular training burns the fat. A combination of both of them will help you reach your goals quicker.

- Do not perform cardiovascular workouts prior to weight training (a 5 to 10-minute warm-up is plenty to elevate body temperature and to get the blood flowing and muscles warmed up). A full cardiovascular workout taps into the glycogen reserves, sugars stored in the muscles that our bodies need to preserve to lift weights. It would be best to perform cardiovascular activities after weight training.

<u>Caloric Intake Formula</u>

Below is a great way to figure out how many calories you need each day to maintain your current weight. Then increase/decrease 250-500 calories depending on your goal.

1. Calculate your Basal Metabolic Rate (BMR) using the Harris-Benedict formula:

Women:
BMR = 655.1 + (4.35 × weight in pounds) + (4.7 × height in inches) - (4.7 × age in years)

Men:
BMR = 66 + (6.2 × weight in pounds) + (12.7 × height in inches) – (6.76 × age in years)

2. Calculate your Total Daily Energy Expenditure (TDEE)

TDEE = BMR × Activity Factor

Enter your BMR into the equation above, then use the table below to plug in your activity factor based on your daily activity level. The TDEE will tell you how many calories you need to eat in order to maintain your current weight.

Amount of Daily Exercise/Activity	Description	Activity Factor
Sedentary	Little or no Exercise/desk job	1.2
Lightly active	Light exercise/sports 1 – 3 days/week	1.375
Moderately active	Moderate Exercise/sports 3 – 5 days/week	1.55
Very active	Heavy Exercise/sports 6 – 7 days/week	1.725
Extremely active	Very heavy exercise/physical job/training 2x/day	1.9

Healthy Food List

Below is the same macronutrient food list presenting good choices for protein, carbohydrates, and fats that were shown in the book. Please feel free to use this as a quick reference rather than needing to page through the book to find the list on the fly.

Proteins

- Beef Tenderloin
- Boneless, Skinless Chicken Breast
 -Egg Whites or Eggs
- Extra Lean Ground Beef or Ground Round
- Eye of Round
- Fish
- Flank Steak
- Ground Turkey, Turkey Breast Slices or Cutlets (fresh sources, not deli cuts)
- Protein Powder
- Ribeye Steaks or Roast
- Shrimp
- Top Round Steaks or Roast
- Top Sirloin
- Top Loin
- Tuna (fresh cut or tuna in can/package with water, not in oil)

Complex Carbs

- Beans (Black, Kidney, Pinto)
- Brown Rice
- Cream of Wheat
- Garbanzo Beans
- Green Peas
- Legumes
- Lentils
- Lima Beans
- Multi-Grain Hot Cereal
- Oat Bran Cereal
- Oatmeal (Old Fashioned or Quick Oats)
- Pasta
- Potatoes (Red or Baking)
- Quinoa
- Rice (White, Jasmine, Wild)
- Sweet Potatoes
- Yams
- Whole-Grains (Bread or Cereal)

Fibrous Carbs

- Asparagus
- Bell Peppers
- Broccoli
- Brussels Sprouts
- Carrots
- Cauliflower
- Celery
- Cucumber
- Egg Plant

- Green Beans
- Green Leafy Lettuce (Green Leaf, Red Leaf, Romaine)
- Kale
- Mushrooms
- Onions
- Peppers (Green or Red)
- Spaghetti Squash
- Spinach
- String Beans
- Zucchini

Fruits

- Apples
- Bananas
- Blueberries
- Grapefruit
- Grapes
- Kiwis
- Oranges
- Papayas
- Raspberries
- Strawberries
- Tomatoes

Healthy Fats

- Fatty Cold-Water Fish (Bluefish, Mackerel, Mullet, Sablefish, Salmon)
- Monounsaturated Oils (Canola, Olive, Peanut)
- More Fish (Anchovy, Herring, Lake Trout,

Sardines, Tuna)
- Natural Almond Butter
- Natural Peanut Butter
- Nuts (Almonds, Peanuts, Pistachios, Walnuts)
- Polyunsaturated Oils (Corn, Cottonseed, Safflower, Soybean, Sunflower)
- Seeds (Flaxseeds, Pumpkin, Sunflower)

Dairy & Eggs

- Eggs (Whole)
- Low-Fat Cottage Cheese
- Low-Fat Yogurt
- Low or Non-Fat Milk

THANK YOU!

I would like to take some time to thank you for reading this book. I truly hope you learned something to help you reach your health and fitness goals. It was a pleasure writing this and my ultimate goal is to help anyone and everyone I can through my work. While some of the information presented was repetitive, it's a great way to embed the information in the human brain and help retain the information and fully grasp what you are reading.

If you found this book helpful, please let me know by going to my website (www.weikfitness.com) and clicking "Contact". I'd love to hear your feedback and if you feel this book would benefit your friends and family, please recommend they too download the book. Thank you again for purchasing and reading my book and I hope it inspires you to go out and live a healthy lifestyle.

"The greatest wealth is health." -- Publius Vergilius Maro (Virgil)

Resources

Anonymous. (2003, April). Exercise and Cancer Prevention [Electronic Version].
Cancer Information Service in the Holden Comprehensive Cancer Center.
Retrieved from http://www.vh.org/adult/patient/cancercenter/cancertips/exercise.html.

Baechle, Thomas R., Earle, Roger W. (2000). *Essentials of Strength Training and Conditioning*. Champaign: Human Kinetics.

Brown, Jean K. (2003). Nutrition and Physical Activity During and After Cancer Treatment: An American Cancer Society Guide for Informed Choices. *CA: A Cancer Journal for Clinician*, 53, 268-291.

Casey, A., D. Constanin-Teodosiu, S. Howell, E. Hultman, and P.L. Greenhaff. Creatine ingestion favorably affects performance and muscle metabolism during maximal exercise in humans. *Am. J. Physiol*. 271: E31-E37. 1996.

Ries LAG, Eisner MP, Kosary CL, et al, eds. SEER Cancer Statistics Review, 1975-

2000. Bethesda, MD: National Cancer
Institute; 2003. Retrieved from
http://seer.cancer.gov/csr/1975-2000.

Savaiano, Dennis. (2000, February). Studies
Confirm Diet and Exercise Are Key in
Cancer Prevention. *Personal MD: Your
Lifeline Online*. Retrieved from
http://www.personalmd.com/news/n02240
14743.shtml.

Shils ME, Olson JA. (1999). *Modern Nutrition in
Health and Disease* (9th Ed.).
Baltimore: Williams & Wilkins.

Terjung, RL et al. (March 2000) American
College of Sports Medicine Roundtable: the
Physiological and Health Effects of Oral
Creatine Supplements. *Medicine and
Science in Sports and Exercise* 32(3):
706-717.

Whitney, Eleanor Noss & Rolfes, Sharon Rady.
(1999). *Understanding Nutrition* (8th
Ed.). Belmont: West/Wadsworth.

Williams, Melvin H. (1998). *The Ergogenics
Edge: Pushing the Limits of Sports
Performance*. Champaign: Human
Kinetics.